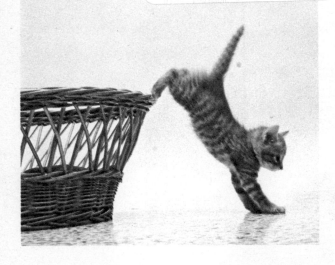

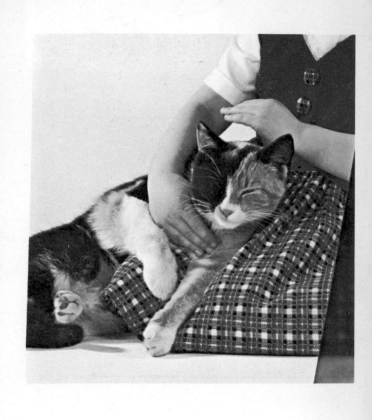

THE Cat YOU CARE FOR

CARE FOR

FELICIA AMES

Director, Friskies Cat Council

With 60 photographs in color by
WALTER CHANDOHA

A SIGNET BOOK from
NEW AMERICAN LIBRARY
TIMES MIRROR

EIGHTH PRINTING

 SIGNET TRADEMARK REG. U.S. PAT. OFF. AND FOREIGN COUNTRIES
REGISTERED TRADEMARK—MARCA REGISTRADA
HECHO EN CHICAGO, U.S.A.

SIGNET, SIGNET CLASSICS, SIGNETTE, MENTOR AND PLUME BOOKS
are published by The New American Library, Inc.,
1301 Avenue of the Americas, New York, New York 10019

FIRST PRINTING, AUGUST, 1968

PRINTED IN THE UNITED STATES OF AMERICA

CONTENTS

9: A Few Feline Fallacies

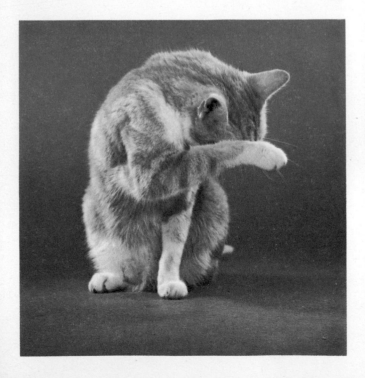

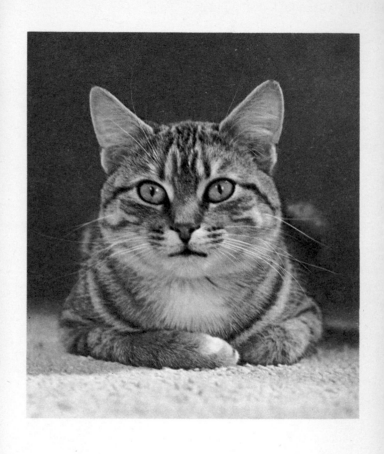

Acknowledgments

This book has been written with the technical assistance of:

Carnation Research Center, Van Nuys, California
  J. M. McIntire, Ph.D., General Manager
  Harry Kimpel, Ph.D., Director, Bio-Med Technical Services
  Lloyd Miller, Ph.D., Manager, Nutrition Research
  Donald B. Morden, Manager, Pet Food Research

Carnation Farms, Carnation, Washington
  Erich Studer, D.V.M., Director, Friskies Research Kennels
  A. H. McDaniel, Ph.D., Associate Director of Research

Robert L. Stansbury, D.V.M., Consultant in Feline Medicine, Carnation Company

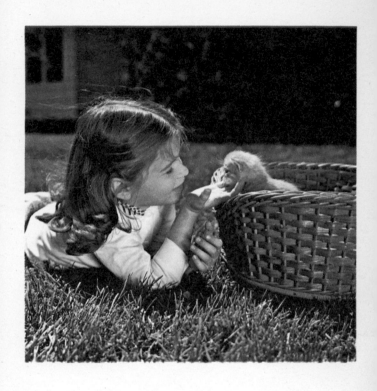

FOREWORD

So now you have a cat.

You've made a wonderful choice of a pet. A cat's quiet grace, mysterious wisdom, intelligence, and perpetual playfulness are a joy to live with.

The cat's hereditary role — which dates back more than five thousand years to ancient Egypt — has always been that of protector of the household and companion to its master. These many years of domesticity have produced an animal that, in spite of its predatory instincts, is meant to be lived with and loved by people. No wonder the cat — so gentle, so unobtrusive, so scrupulously clean — fits so naturally into home life.

Although the cat's independent personality makes him appear self-sufficient, he is totally dependent on you for proper care and, equally important, for love.

But loving care needs knowledge to make it intelligent care. Friskies hopes that this book can give you the know-how to take on this new responsibility with pleasure and ease.

Read and refer to this little book often. And may your cat have a long and happy life.

1

Now That There's A Cat In Your Life

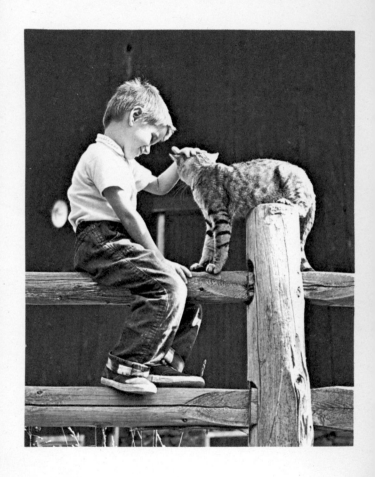

How to Tell a Cat from a Dog

Except for the fact that a cat is a four-footed, furry domestic animal, you should find little resemblance between a cat and a dog. The sooner you discern this fact the better.

The relationship you have with a cat is entirely different from the one you have with a dog. A dog will go all out to win your favor — the cat is not even remotely interested in doing something just to please you. (If you are happy with him, that's *your* doing, not his!)

In spite of this seemingly self-centered approach to life, the cat is a very loving animal; he craves your affection and attention, but he wants it on his own terms. You train a dog. A cat thinks obeying commands somewhat beneath his dignity. A dog's personality varies with the breed. Each cat is a true individual, regardless of breed. His charm lies in the fact that no cat is like any other, and all are full of surprises.

Most cats want to be near you, but they don't fawn over you. They treat you as an equal. You can always be the center of a dog's world; you will never be the center of a cat's world. Unlike a dog, who is a born joiner, a cat is a born loner. He is self-possessed, knows exactly what he wants and where he is going. Independent? Yes. But independent in the sense of being mature, not indifferent.

You appreciate a dog for his responsiveness to you — a cat for his beauty, grace, and intelligence, combined with subtle signs of affection.

So before you adopt a cat, be sure you don't want a cat that acts like a dog. There is no such animal.

Before You Take Your Cat Home

It's easy to fall in love with a kitten. But before you get carried away with that furry ball of fun, be sure you are up to the responsibility of lifetime care.

Give these points some thought before you adopt your kitten:

• Remember that little kittens soon grow into large cats, with hair that sheds and claws that sometimes shred. Will you love kitty then?

• Are you prepared to meet the expense of proper diet (not just scraps), inoculations, and altering? (Both female *and* male cats should be altered if you want a satisfactory pet.)

• Are you willing to take your pet to a veterinarian for proper care when he is ill or injured?

• Do you know the laws of your community governing the humane treatment of animals and their control?

• Do you really *like* cats? If the personality of a grown cat makes you nervous, you'd better think about another choice of pet.

Why not take two — they're small

Think about taking home a *pair* of cats or kittens. They can be more than twice the fun — and hardly more care than one. Two kittens romping, wrestling, and snoozing together are a delight to watch. They'll exercise better and, of course, keep each other constant company. Your lone cat will be much more dependent on you.

Long-hair or short?

That fluffy Persian kitten may be irresistible, but remember that the cat can't take care of that luxurious coat all by himself. You *must* comb a long-haired cat daily or he will soon be a mass of tangles and mats.

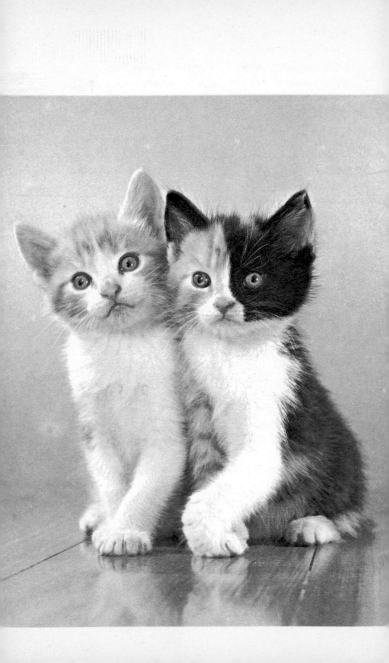

Is anyone in your family allergic to cat hair? It makes some people sniffle. Some sneezers can live with short-haired cats, but the long-hairs send them into near fits.

Male or female?

Male cats are more aggressive, independent, and tend to be roamers. They are, however, just as affectionate as females. Males often grow to a larger size than females. The female is a bit quieter (except in season), more passive, and home-loving.

Here's how you can tell the sex of the cat. Underneath the tail on males you see a period (.), on females, an upside down exclamation mark (¡). You need not be concerned about the sex of your cat if you plan to have it altered (see page 67). Either sex makes an equally lovable pet.

Prepare for the ride home

Most cats (until conditioned, anyway) don't like automobiles. If you don't wish to drive with a cat clawing at your shoulder, you had better provide a container for the ride home. (A frightened kitten may scratch the person who is trying to hold it.) A very deep carton will do for a small kitten.

It might be a good idea to purchase your cat carrier right now. You'll find it most handy for taking your cat to the veterinarian, even if you don't plan to take kitty on any other trips. (See page 77 on carriers.)

Introducing the New Pet

Let the cat's first day at home be a quiet one. He should be allowed peace and freedom to get acquainted with his new surroundings. Handle the newcomer as little as possible (easier said than done!), and keep the children from frightening poor kitty with their joyful enthusiasm.

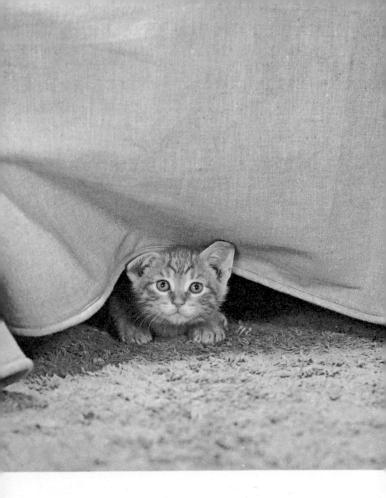

Introduce other pets slowly

Keep the dog and cat apart, perhaps even for several days, until they are well aware of each other's scent. Make their first meetings short. *Don't* feed them together. You should not leave the pets alone together until you see definite signs of affection.

If you have another cat, give him no chance to be jealous of the newcomer. Introduce them in the same slow manner as you would a dog, keeping them

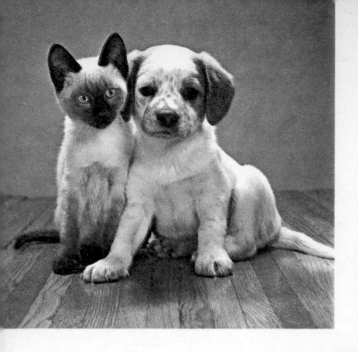

apart until they are well aware of each other's presence. Show extra affection to the older member whenever the newcomer is present. Eventually the older cat will probably take a parental and protective attitude toward the younger and be pleased to have a new friend.

If you use a cautious introductory technique, your cat, especially if he is a kitten, can become friends with almost any animal — the pet white rat, the bird, the rabbit. And what amusing friends they make! Let the cat make the first overtures; don't just throw them together. If Puss has a place to climb, he will feel safer and hence less afraid of the other animal. (See page 118 on cats and their friends.)

Handle kitty gently, *always*

Be gentle and avoid loud or sudden noises. Be sure that everyone who has the urge to pick up the new pet knows how to do so properly. Constant frightening and mishandling of a kitten can quickly make it defensive and unfriendly.

Don't pick up a kitten or cat by the nape of the neck. Neck-dangling is painful and can cause injury. Instead, place one hand under the cat's body, just behind the front legs; with the other hand, brace the hind feet. Your cat feels secure this way.

A Cat Belongs in the House (Most of the Time)

Decide now where the cat is to have his quarters. Unless he is supposed to keep mice out of the barn, you should house him inside.

The cat likes his living warm, cozy, and sunny; the garage, shed, or basement just won't do. (Remember, the cat is independent — if accommodations aren't to his liking, he may just pick up and move!)

Prepare a bed

You can buy your cat a fancy bed, or you can line a cardboard box with a washable blanket. He will like

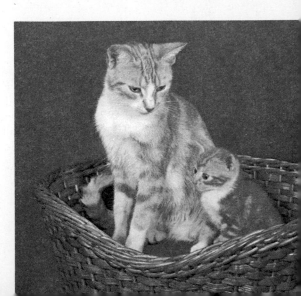

his bed if it is soft, warm, free from drafts, and off the floor. Cats have a perching instinct and prefer to sleep *up*. Be sure to change your cat's bedding as often as you would your own. He's as fastidious as you are.

After you've prepared kitty a nice bed, don't be hurt if he chooses to sleep somewhere else. Just spread a towel over the favored spot and let him have his way.

Fix a litterbox

Cats are so wonderfully clean that they will housebreak themselves if given half a chance. Line an enamel or plastic pan (large enough for the cat to turn around in) with newspapers; add a small amount of sand or absorbent litter material (available at markets and pet stores). Put the new kitten in the fresh sand and show him how to paw it. If the litter box is kept where your cat can locate it quickly, you will find that he uses it consistently right from the start. If you have a large house, use two or three pans.

Keep the box clean. Change the litter material frequently, preferably every time it is used; a soiled litterbox is offensive to the cat and can cause disease. Wash the litter pan with soap and water each time you change the filler, and sterilize with a laundry bleach. Be sure to rinse thoroughly after sterilizing. Kitty doesn't like that smell!

If you have a home with a yard, you may have your cat use the litterbox only when he is confined to the house — but always provide one.

A collar is a good idea

A collar tagged with your name and address protects your cat against loss. If the collar has a bell, it's a bird warning, though some cats are so smart they can walk without ringing the bell. You'll want your cat collared if you plan to leash-walk him.

If the collar is introduced to the kitten early enough, he probably will not object to it. If you use a leather

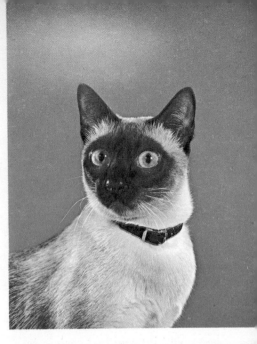

strap, be sure it is loose enough to slip over the head in case your cat gets caught on a tree branch. (An elasticized safety collar eliminates this danger.)

If you have put a collar on your kitten, check frequently to be sure it fits loosely. That kitten grows especially fast when you're not looking.

Provide a scratching post

All cats need to scratch. Therefore, all cats need a scratching post — unless you're willing to donate your good sofa to the cause.

You can make a good scratching post by nailing a piece of old carpet (under which you've placed some catnip) to a post. If kitty starts to scratch your furniture, give him a firm and loud "No!" Then show him how to use his post by running his claws down it. (A spring toy attached to the top of the post makes it even more attractive.)

Don't wait until the cat starts clawing the furniture. You'll have better luck if you get him started on the

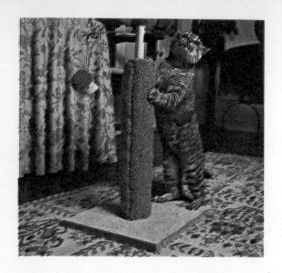

post right away. He may never find out that the sofa is another possibility.

If the cat prefers the sofa to the post, discourage him by tying a bag of moth balls behind the sofa back. (Commercial repellents seem to do little good.) For complete peace of mind, shut the cat out of the room when you're not there to say "No!"

If clawing becomes a serious problem, and if your cat is an indoor cat, ask your veterinarian about safe removal of the *front* claws. (Even an outdoor cat can still defend himself with his hind feet, and can still climb a tree.) This is definitely a last resort, but better to lose the claws than to give up the cat.

Shopping for Your Cat's Needs

Devote a shopping trip to getting all your cat's needs the first day so that he will truly feel at home from then on. Suggested are:

- Litter pan(s) and absorbent litter
- Collar and identification tag

- Toys — such as catnip mouse, hard rubber ball, rubber mouse, ping-pong or other plastic balls
- Non-tippable, rustproof food and water bowls
- Cat carrier (one that opens from the top and is covered on the sides is preferable)
- Scratching post (if you decide not to make one)
- Grooming aids (see page 33)
- Supply of food (see pages 41 - 47)
- First aid needs (see page 62)

Tips on Safety

Felines are canny and careful — but even so, you must be on the alert for your cat's safety.

Cat-proof the outdoors

Don't let your new kitten out in the yard alone until you've checked the fence for holes. Go through the garage and basement, putting away poisons and paints. Don't keep mouse or rat traps where the cat might walk into them. Clear the premises of toxic rat or roach poisons and insecticides.

Is a cat safe in a tree?

Many cat owners panic the first time Puss gets up and out on a tree limb, a long way above the hard ground. And no wonder. Puss panics too, and his howls

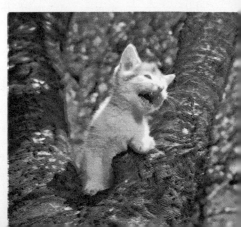

are pathetic. Consequently, Dad must play Tarzan, and risk his own and the tree's limbs; or Mother must play helpless and call the fire department.

The surest, safest cure for a cat with high ambitions is to leave him alone, heartless though it may seem at the time, says Robert Lothar Kendell, head of the American Feline Society since 1938. The Newtonian principle that what goes up will come down holds true for cats, too, although it sometimes takes a bit of time. Coaxing and calling will only make kitty more nervous about his precarious position. "No cat has ever fallen out of a tree," states Mr. Kendell. "And as far as I know, no cat ever starved to death in a tree."*

Inside the house there's danger, too

Remember, cats are curious. Don't leave tubs filled with water when there's a kitten in the house. He may investigate by walking around the edge of the tub. First thing you know — kersplash! Keep the toilets closed. Screen all high windows. Flatten dangerous tin cans, and keep sharp can lids out of kitty's way. Put the sewing basket out of reach. Threads and yarns can be swallowed — so much the worse if a needle is attached.

Shut all cupboards and drawers (but check first to make sure that kitty isn't inside). Don't leave the clothes dryer open — cats have been tumble-dried to death.

Kitty loves dangling cords. Make sure he doesn't yank down the iron, the electric skillet, the toaster, or the percolator. And don't let him chew cords to see what might be inside. What's inside is Big Trouble.

Christmas is an especially dangerous time

As you herald in the holiday season, take care that kitty's first Noel won't be his last. The cat's delight with the tree will be obvious. Keep him away from

*"How To Get a Cat Out of a Tree," *Changing Times*, May 1967.

it entirely if you can. Broken ornaments can perforate an intestine, swallowed tinsel can cause intestinal blockage, artificial snow is poisonous, and cotton is almost as bad.

Keep Puss away from the unwrapping of presents, too. He would love to make a meal of ribbon, cord, and string — resulting in painful constipation. Even worse, swallowed string or ribbon can become tightly embedded in the loops of the bowel and cause perforating ulcers. As for mistletoe, hang it high! It's poisonous for the cat.

Danger walks at night

If you love kitty, keep him in after sundown, even though he'd so enjoy the hunt at night. Cars are probably the number one cat-killer in the United States, and while a nimble cat usually manages to dodge a car in daylight, headlights may cause him to "freeze" in the middle of the road, where he helplessly awaits sudden death.

Fighting is another nighttime hazard. Probably more cat injuries are received in fights with cats, dogs, or other animals than from any accidental cause, and most fights take place at night.

How to stop a cat fight

When you're called by loud yowls to witness a cat fight, *don't* let them fight it out. Serious injuries can

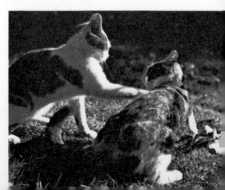

result — those cats mean business. Don't try "shooing" — it won't work. Don't try to pull the cats away from each other — you'll end up with *your* paws bandaged (see page 57 on cat bites). A bucket of water splashed in the middle of the ruckus will usually break it up. Or, if your aim is bad, try the hose.

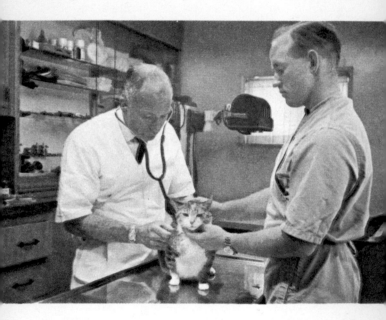

Health Precautions Are a Must

At your first opportunity, take your cat to a veterinarian for a checkup and necessary inoculations.

Shots for infectious enteritis

Infectious enteritis, or panleukopenia (also known as cat fever, and sometimes erroneously called cat distemper), is highly contagious and the most deadly of cat diseases (see page 51). Two shots, administered a week apart when the kitten is seven to nine weeks old, are mandatory if you want him to escape this dread and nearly always fatal disease. A single enteritis shot is sometimes used, but is generally not recommended for the greatest immunity. Many veterinarians also advise shots against rabies and pneumonitis.

Finding a veterinarian

When you have your cat inoculated is a good time to find a veterinarian whom you feel you can turn to with confidence in an emergency. It is a wise idea to inquire if there is a twenty-four-hour emergency veterinary service in your area and to keep its telephone number handy.

You will know immediately by the way the veterinarian handles your animal whether or not he likes cats and will take a real interest in your pet's health. Some veterinarians specialize in cats. The interested veterinarian will be glad to discuss any questions you have about cat care and feeding and will warn you about other diseases which might endanger your pet.

2

Grooming Shows
You Care

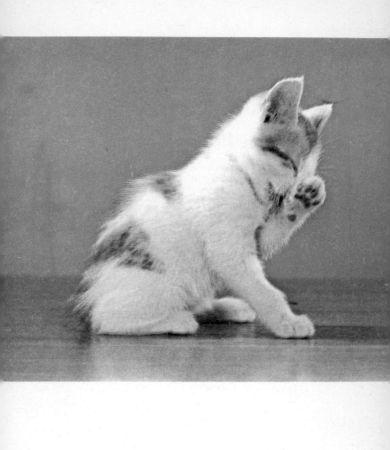

Grooming Aids

After watching how meticulously your cat takes care of himself, you may feel that grooming your cat is like gilding the lily. But even these frequent cat tongue-baths are not quite enough.

For proper grooming you will need:
- Brush, with bristles long and strong enough to do a good job (for short-haired cats)
- Steel comb (for long-haired cats)
- Flea comb
- Nail clippers made especially for cats
- Baby oil or hydrogen peroxide
- Cotton swab sticks

Daily Brushing and Combing

Short-hair or long-hair, show cat or pet cat, your feline should have a daily brushing or combing to keep the hairs off the furniture and the fleas off the cat. Just a few minutes a day will assure your cat a handsome coat, limit shedding, discourage fleas, and prevent hair balls.

Begin grooming when the cat is still a kitten — as early as two weeks — so he will become accustomed to the routine. Brush or comb, gently and quickly, with the grain. Combing is especially necessary for long-haired cats. Use a strong metal comb. If a long-haired coat becomes too matted, you may have to cut the tangle. Use small scissors. Point them outward and cut with the hair, not across it.

Bathing

With daily brushing and combing, bathing a cat

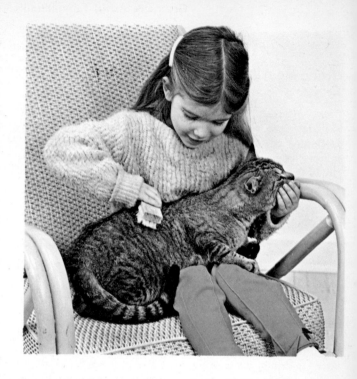

is an emergency measure only, unless, of course, you have a show cat. Pedigreed cats are always bathed and groomed before shows. When the necessity does arise, use only warm water and mild soap (no detergent). There are a number of good cat shampoos available. You may put a drop of white petroleum jelly in the corner of each of his eyes to keep the suds out.

The best method for bathing is to use two tubs or a double sink so that you can dunk and rinse quickly. Rinse the cat thoroughly and dry well with towels; then keep him warm and out of drafts until he is thoroughly fluffed out again. (Cats catch cold easily.)

Do not bathe a kitten under six months of age. Some cat owners find that a dry bath of talcum powder, corn meal, or dry shampoo is a very satisfactory answer to the cat-bathing problem.

Clipping

Should cats be clipped in summer?

The sight of a cat up to its ears in fur in mid-July is enough to send some owners to the veterinarian with a plea to clip or thin the coat. Authorities differ on this point, but it seems to be the best veterinary opinion to leave the coat alone. Clipping is often humiliating for a cat; it may cause psychological trauma much more unbearable than the heat. You'll be doing your cat a greater kindness during the summer (when he is shedding heavily) if you brush or comb him frequently and then leave him alone to rest himself lazily in his favorite cool spot.

Whiskers

Since they serve as a cat's antennae, whiskers are a vital part of his sensory equipment. You probably

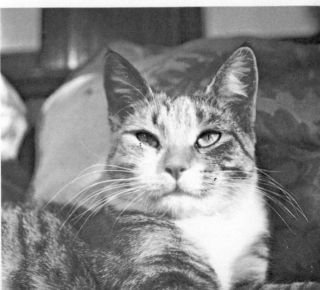

know better than to clip them, but be sure to keep the children from playing "barber shop" with the cat.

Nail clipping

If your cat spends most of his time indoors, you may have to clip his claws occasionally. His paws will become uncomfortable if the nails are not worn down. Nail clipping will not prevent him from doing his scratching exercises, nor will it prevent him from climbing safely. Use only clippers made especially for cat claws (such as Resco), and trim only the slightest bit of the nail. Claws should be clipped when introducing the cat to a dog and before entering him in a cat show.

Ears

The cat ordinarily keeps his ears clean, but you may wish to cleanse them with a cotton swab stick moistened with baby oil or hydrogen peroxide when you are checking for ear mites. Never go deeper than you can see. Ear mites, which look like small black specks resembling coffee grounds, can cause your cat much grief and should be treated promptly (see page 56 on mites).

Teeth

Kittens cut their second teeth when they are from two to six months of age. Large bones or kibbles (Little Friskies) are appealing to the teething kitten, but no chicken or chop bones, please. They can splinter and cause real trouble.

You should check your cat's teeth regularly for evidence of eroded enamel or accumulated tartar and have your veterinarian treat these conditions. If your cat is occasionally given a large bone to chew on, tartar deposits can sometimes be prevented.

Eyes

A healthy cat's eyes are bright and clear. They usually require no care, unless illness, such as a cold, causes mucus to accumulate. Then you may wash kitty's eyes with a mild solution of warm salt water.

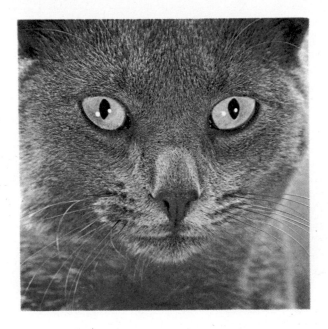

3

Food That Keeps Him Happy

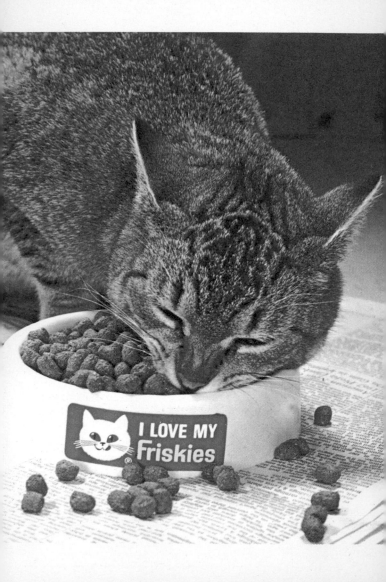

FEEDING your cat the right amounts of the proper foods is all-important to growth, appearance, vitality, and long life.

How Much?

Unless they have been starved or have become accustomed to being overfed, cats are fairly sensible about their food and will eat only the amounts they need. Don't tempt Puss to eat more by leaving the food dish out. When he turns away from it and starts his after-meal tidy-up, that's your signal to remove the food. It is impossible to say flatly how much a cat should eat. Needs vary depending on the cat's age, size, activity, and temperament. But it is always safer to underfeed rather than to overfeed your cat. He'll tell you in no uncertain terms when you're being too stingy with the rations!

How Often?

Kittens need to be fed frequently, at least four times a day. As the kitten grows, decrease the number of meals while increasing the amount of each feeding.

By seven months your cat will have his permanent teeth. You may then cut the feedings down to three or even two times a day. A full-grown cat needs to eat only twice daily — morning and night. (Some full-grown cats are not aware of this fact, however, and insist on lunch, too. Others do very well on just one meal a day.)

It is important to preserve routine in feeding a cat. Always feed at the same time and in the same place. Cats like to take their food out of the dish, so be prepared — always place the food dish on a newspaper. (Some cats even eat with their paws, and are left- or right-pawed from birth.)

Water

There should always be plenty of fresh water in the cat's drinking dish. Change the water daily, and in hot weather, oftener. Even if you never *see* your cat drink water, he does. A clean water dish will discourage him from drinking out of the toilet bowl, flower dish, or fish tank!

What About Milk?

Contrary to common belief, adult cats do not need, and often don't like, milk. While a few seem to thrive on it, for many more it causes diarrhea. Your small kitten should have either fresh or evaporated milk, such as Carnation, mixed with his food, one tablespoon to a feeding. Your kitten's feedings may be supplemented gradually with as much milk as he will drink, *after* the solid food has been given. In general, however, milk is not a "must" for most mature cats, unless they seem to crave it and no intestinal upset occurs. Their calcium needs are met by a quality commercial cat food, and by occasional treats of cottage cheese, a food they love.

What To Feed?

More important than the amounts fed are the *kinds* of food your cat eats. A *well-balanced* diet is necessary — for health, disposition, beauty. The proper diet for a cat must contain proteins, fat, and vitamins and minerals, in the correct proportions.

You can be sure that your cat obtains all these essentials by feeding him a regular diet of a quality commercial cat food, such as Friskies. Of the many brands of pet food on the market today, only a few have been formulated through careful scientific research to provide a balanced diet for your cat day after day.

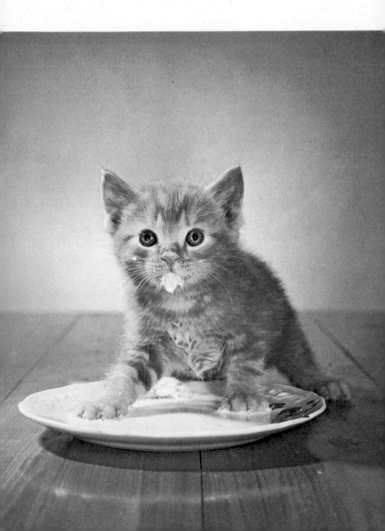

Your cat will enjoy an occasional serving of fresh raw meat, such as horse meat, beef, or lamb kidney, melts, or raw liver, but fresh meats are not necessary for a balanced diet. Too much liver has a laxative effect. Fish should always be cooked, and raw pork-muscle meat avoided entirely. Raw pork liver and heart are acceptable; pork kidney less so. Cats should *not* be fed a diet of lean meat exclusively or they will suffer deficiency symptoms.

Once you have found a fully balanced diet (be sure to check the label for vitamin content) you should stay with one brand (but not one flavor); diet changes, unless done gradually, can be upsetting.

Finicky eater or gourmet?

Some cat fanciers get a little too fancy — they take pride in the fact that their Puss will eat only caviar and cream, or some such nonsense. These exotic tastes only develop because the doting owners have conditioned the cat to like such expensive foods. Any cat can and should be trained to eat a reasonable diet. Tempting him with table delicacies can cause your cat to overeat, or fill his tummy so that he does not relish the balanced diet you provide for him.

On the other hand, a cat, unlike a dog, *is* something of an epicure. Most dogs will gobble almost anything set in front of them. A cat approaches a meal with caution, sniffs at it delicately to be sure it is on his preferred list, and only then takes a bite. If he doesn't care for the offering that day, he will look at the dish with obvious scorn and walk away hungry.

Variety? Yes!

Ask any cat and he will tell you that variety in his menu is basic cat courtesy, although not nutritionally necessary. Even liver, if offered day after day, can become a real bore.

Cat owners are often surprised to find that their

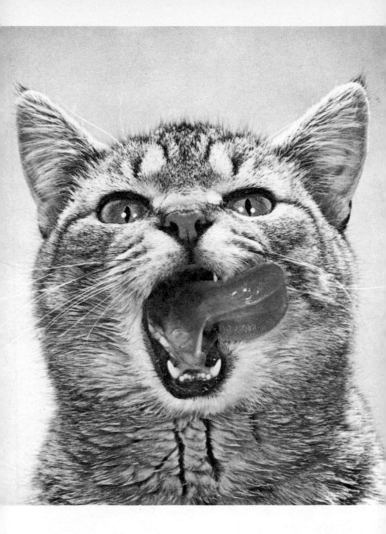

carnivorous pet has a taste for vegetables — especially peas, string beans, and asparagus. Some cats have been known to hanker for olives, mushrooms, and even artichokes. If you'd like to know what foods your Puss has a tooth for, just keep an eye on what he tries to snitch (and even the most well-mannered cats *do* snitch.)

Speaking of snitching, you'll be wise to defrost your frozen foods, especially meats, on a shelf that's "unleapable," or your dinner may disappear. The unwarmed oven is a good place; then Puss doesn't even get a whiff.

Whether or not you serve your cat vegetables, he does need some fresh greenery to chew on occasionally. If he's a house cat, plant a little flower pot with grass seed and let him have his own pasture. Cats also like ferns, petunias, nasturtiums, and marigolds. Occasional nibbles are good for them (if not for the garden).

Giving Your Cat a Choice

Thanks to research carried on for many years at Carnation Company's pet facilities, both at the Research Laboratories, Van Nuys, California, and at Carnation Farms, Washington, any or all of these pet foods provide a completely nourishing diet for your cat — the best nutrition modern science has been able to devise.

Little Friskies Dry Cat Food—Ocean Fish, Country Chicken, Braised Liver, Tuna, Seafood, Giblets & Liver flavors

Friskies Canned Cat Food—Fish, Chicken, Liver, Kidney, Meat flavors

Friskies Cat Food Buffet—in fifteen combinations, such as Chicken, Fish & Liver, Liver & Chicken, Giblets & Turkey, Mixed Grill, Dixie Dinner

Some Feeding Don'ts

• Don't feed your cat cold food — bring it to room temperature. Cold food can cause diarrhea and vomiting. Cold milk on a hot day can make kittens very sick. And they don't like it cold anyway.

• Don't substitute milk for water, or milk for a meal of solid food. Milk has a laxative effect on many cats and should be given sparingly, *after* a meal, if at all. If you use evaporated milk, dilute it a little with warm water.

• Don't leave kitty's food out in the bowl. The food will spoil, and you will also spoil kitty, who will soon expect food at all hours. An important exception is nourishing dry food, such as Little Friskies, which may be left out for snacking or for times when you have to be away. The cat will eat only as much as he needs at each meal. (The texture of dry food is good for Puss's teeth, too.)

• Don't add mineral oil to food. Mineral oil interferes with vitamin absorption. If oil is administered to make the coat shiny, use vegetable oil such as corn or safflower oil.

• Don't feed your cat raw fresh-water fish. It contains thiaminase, an enzyme that destroys some of the B vitamins.

• Don't cut down on kitty's rations to make him a good hunter. Starving him will just keep him so weak that he couldn't bag a mouse if it were tied up with a ribbon.

• Don't feed your cat small or sharp bones (such as chicken bones). They can splinter and cause choking, or pierce the stomach and intestinal walls.

• Don't disturb your pet while he is eating. He has a one-track mind and a sensitive nervous system.

• Don't feed your cat a mono-diet. If *you* are tired of roast beef by the time it is hash, think how your cat feels.

• And finally, don't feed a cat as you would a human being. Feed him like a cat.

4

What Ails That Cat ?

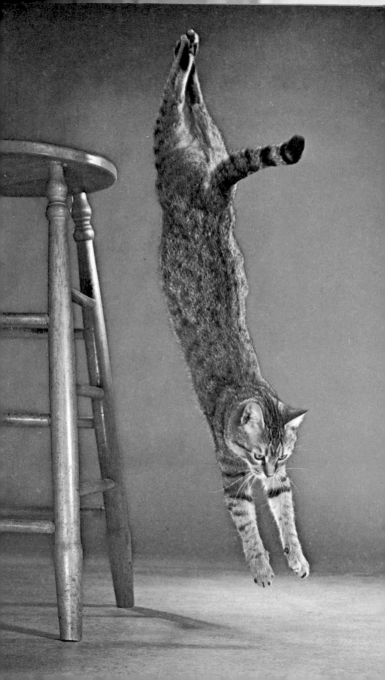

YOU instinctively know when your cat is healthy. He's alert and full of fun; his coat glistens, his eyes sparkle. When he becomes ill, you may notice the following changes:

- Dull, rough coat, excessive shedding
- Listlessness, sleepiness
- Bad breath
- Refusal of food
- Eyes that are dull, watery, red
- Appearance of the "third eyelid," or film, over a period of time (usually indicating intestinal difficulty)
- Vomiting, coughing, sneezing
- Acute swelling, or lumps which increase in size

At any of these danger signals, take your cat's temperature and call your veterinarian. A cat doesn't malinger. If he acts a *little* sick, chances are he may be *very* sick.

Common Ailments

Study the following descriptions of common ailments that plague cats and familiarize yourself with their symptoms. Many of the ailments can be avoided by proper, watchful care.

Infectious enteritis (or panleukopenia)

Mistakenly called feline distemper, it is nearly always fatal to kittens; the mortality rate with older cats is only a little more favorable. Fortunately, this disease is not the threat it once was; kittens as young as seven to nine weeks can be immunized effectively.

Symptoms of the disease vary. They are sudden and violent. Treatment is lengthy and expensive for the few cats that do survive. Therapy includes blood transfusions, antibiotics, and fluids. Early vaccination is a must (see page 28).

Viro-rhinotracheitis (or flu)

Cat flu resembles the common cold in humans. The runny nose and eyes, sneezing, and occasional fever that accompany it can make your cat uncomfortable for a few days. Keep him indoors and out of drafts. If symptoms persist, take him to the veterinarian. It may be pneumonitis.

Pneumonitis

A severe disease of the upper respiratory tract, its early symptoms are much the same as those of rhinotracheitis, but more severe — fever, sneezing, runny eyes, wheezing, drooling. Given proper treatment with antibiotics, most cats recover in two to three weeks. Many veterinarians recommend annual inoculations against pneumonitis, although there are so many viruses which can cause it that it is almost impossible to immunize successfully.

While infectious enteritis, rhinotracheitis, and pneumonitis are all highly contagious among the feline population, they cannot be transmitted to people.

Rabies

Cats are not as likely to contract rabies as dogs are, but when they do it is always fatal. The disease can be transmitted from a rabid cat to human beings or to other animals. Many veterinarians recommend early rabies vaccination for your cat.

Infectious anemia (hemobartinella)

This virulent disease is on the rise. A parasite, possibly carried by fleas, gets in the blood stream and attacks the red blood cells. Symptoms are loss of appetite, listlessness, and pale mucous membranes. Fatal to more than 51 per cent of all cats that contract it, it can be treated with steroids, antibiotics, and blood transfusions. Prompt veterinary attention is imperative. Too often, unfortunately, treatment is delayed, and the condition deteriorates into leukemia, which is not curable. Since the parasite requires an intermediate host, infectious anemia is not directly contagious — either to other cats or to human beings.

Urolithiasis

Urinary difficulties are common in cats, especially in altered males. If your cat strains in his pan, he may be suffering from any one of a variety of urinary problems rather than from simple constipation. When a cat retains urine due to inability to void, he is in danger of succumbing to uremic poisoning. Urinary problems must always be taken care of promptly by the veterinarian. He may prescribe distilled water, improved sanitary facilities, and/or medication. If these fail to improve the condition, surgery may be indicated.

Hairballs

Because all cats lick themselves clean, they can develop hairballs from swallowed hair. This is, of course, particularly true of long-haired cats. Most often these indigestible lumps are vomited or eliminated through the bowels.

If you suspect, however, that your cat is constipated because of a hairball, you may help him with a tablet of milk of magnesia or one Carter's pill. Another remedy is a dab of white petroleum jelly, about the size of your thumb, placed on the roof of the cat's mouth.

A large hairball can make your cat very ill. Its removal usually requires the assistance of a veterinarian, and may even involve surgery. Daily combing and brushing will remove much of the cat's loose hair, and is, therefore, the best prevention against hairballs.

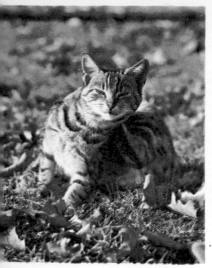
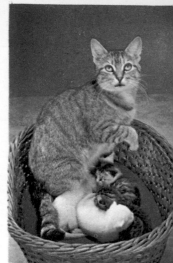

Fleas

These common parasites cause not only itching and scratching but also allergies and anemias, and are a source of worms. Keep your cat's bed immaculate to be sure it does not become a nest for flea eggs.

A flea comb dipped in alcohol, stroked against the direction of the hair, will eliminate many of the pests. Be sure you wet the comb before each stroke.

An aerosol spray which gets right down to the skin is the best flea killer. Ask your veterinarian to recommend one. If your cat protests the sound of the spray too much (sometimes it frightens him), try wetting your hand with the liquid and rubbing it thoroughly into the fur.

Be sure the flea remedy you use is recommended for *cats* — others may be harmful. Even the dog's powder or spray may not be safe for kitty. DDT powders and sprays are lethal for cats.

Recent nutritional research tells us that a diet high in thiamine (one of the B vitamins) will keep a cat free of fleas. A good source of thiamine is brewer's yeast. About a half teaspoonful sprinkled over his food every meal may be a good flea insurance. (Even if your cat doesn't have fleas, he'll probably relish it, and it's very good for him.)

Fleas in the house

Sometimes in hot weather fleas drop off the cat and breed in the corners or carpets. An inexpensive aerosol bomb, available from your veterinarian, will eliminate

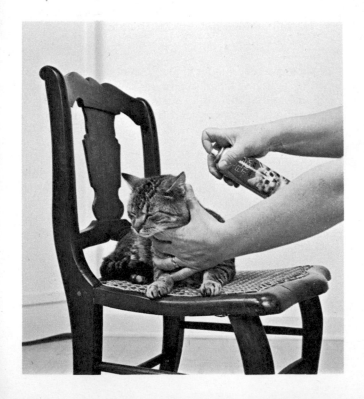

them in a few hours. Some people also use naphthalene flakes in the vacuum cleaner bag to rid their carpets of fleas.

Ear troubles

When dust, dirt, and wax collect in the cat's ear, they provide a breeding ground for bacterial, fungal, and ear mite infections. The best prevention is cleanliness. If your cat paws his ear or shakes his head violently, he has an ear irritation. If it does not clear up after a few days of cleansing with baby oil or hydrogen peroxide on a cotton swab stick (going only as far as you can see), you'll need a veterinarian's help. *Never probe in your cat's ear with a sharp instrument or hairpin.* The only thing you'll find is trouble.

Worms

Worms are heralded by many symptoms — loss of appetite, diarrhea, vomiting, rough coat, loss of weight, or bloated stomach. Call your veterinarian for advice on worming. Do *not* attempt to use a worm remedy without his say-so.

Skin problems

The most common skin problems are eczema, ringworm, and allergy. They can cause your cat's skin to become sore and flaky, and the coat patchy. Sores can spread rapidly. Because there are so many different causes and cures for skin diseases, you should have your veterinarian diagnose and treat the ailment. Don't neglect a skin disease. Nothing can be more irritating to a cat, nor more demoralizing.

Bites, cuts, and scratches

Ordinarily, you need not treat cuts and scratches. The cat will clean them by licking. If too much licking is keeping the wound open, trim the hair, apply a healing ointment (such as Panalog, by Squibb), and then bandage the injured part. Where no bandage is used, be sure to apply a nonpoisonous ointment (*not* zinc oxide or carbolated petroleum jelly).

If a cat bites you

Cat bites or deep claw marks carry with them the danger of blood poisoning. Squeeze the wound to make it bleed as much as possible. Then cleanse it thoroughly with hydrogen peroxide and paint the wound with an antiseptic (ST 37 is good), leaving it open to heal. If the wound is a puncture wound, see your physician as soon as possible to avoid severe infection.

Abscesses

Cat wounds frequently abscess because they are often punctures from animal bites, thorns, or imbedded glass. These wounds do not bleed freely enough to cleanse themselves. Abscesses are accompanied by fever and can be dangerous. Have the veterinarian treat any wound that does not heal promptly.

Diarrhea

Common in cats, diarrhea may be caused by worms, may signal the onset of any number of illnesses, or may merely indicate a minor digestive upset. Too much raw liver or milk can also cause loose stools.

You may treat diarrhea with a light, simple diet, or you may wish to withhold food entirely. Feed raw kidney, heart, or hamburger, and give one teaspoon Kaopectate or Pepto Bismol three times a day. If the diarrhea persists for more than a day or two, notify your veterinarian. It could mean trouble.

Constipation

A rounded teaspoon of white vaseline, one teaspoon of milk of magnesia or one Carter's pill, or an infant's suppository will help constipation. Petromalt or a similar cat remedy, supplemented with vitamins, may also be recommended by your veterinarian.

If these remedies do not help, give the cat an enema of one teaspoon glycerine mixed with three tablespoons warm water. Inject into rectum with infant's bulb-type ear syringe. (It's a good idea to have a second person help you with this procedure.)

Frequent trips to the sand tray may indicate urinary retention, not constipation (See Urolithiasis page 53.)

Eye irritations
Wash with mild, warm salt-water solution.

Poisoning
Symptoms of poisoning include trembling, twitching, shallow breathing, vomiting, convulsions, blood-streaked diarrhea. Call the veterinarian *immediately*. The cat's life will depend on prompt medical attention. The antidote will vary with the type of poison.

If possible, give an emetic right away — hydrogen peroxide mixed with an equal amount of tepid water, salt water (two teaspoons salt to a cup of warm water), or mustard powder (one teaspoon to a cup of tepid water).

Hot weather problems
Heat prostration most often occurs in old cats and fat cats. The cat will appear to pant rapidly, salivate, and, if conscious, have an anxious facial expression. In severe cases treatment has to be immediate; temperatures above 107° Fahrenheit cause brain damage. Treatment consists of sponging the animal in cool water or placing him in a bath that is 60° to 70° Fahrenheit. The progress of the treatment can be checked by frequent rectal temperature checks. If the cat is conscious, small amounts of water should be offered frequently. Call your veterinarian if kitty doesn't snap back quickly.

You can go a long way toward preventing heat pros-

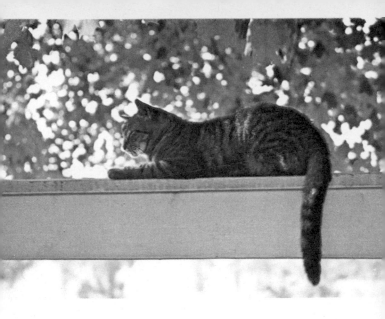

tration by making sure your cat has a dark, shady spot to rest outside in warm weather, or by keeping him indoors. Let him seek out that cool spot on the tile, in the basement, or even in the empty bathtub.

A word of caution. Never cool an overheated cat by feeding him cold milk or water. Ice-cold drinks can cause convulsions. Cool, yes. Cold, no.

Taking the Temperature

Fever is one of the most accurate indicators of illness. If you suspect that your cat is ailing, take his temperature. Insert rectal thermometer, lubricated with white vaseline, so that bulb tip is covered (about half the length). Hold in place for one to three minutes. Normal temperature is about 101.6° Fahrenheit.

Administering Medicines

Don't doctor the cat's food with medication. The sick cat's appetite will probably be off anyway, and he will not eat suspicious tasting food. Consequently, both food and medicine will be wasted.

You may need help to administer the medicine, using restraint on the cat's forelegs.

Restraint for treatment

Restraint is often necessary when giving first aid or medication to a cat. Methods of securing the cat's legs vary with the area to be treated.

1. When treating the head or neck, wrap the cat's body in a heavy bath towel or place the cat in a small laundry bag with the drawstring tightened around his neck. (Be careful not to choke him!)

2. For treatment below the neck, wrap the forelimbs together and the hind limbs together with several turns of a soft bandage.

3. Undoubtedly the best method of immobilization for treatment (provided the treatment is not extremely frightening or painful for the cat) is restraint by another person. This is easily done by holding forepaws together and back paws together — very *firmly* — with the two hands. If the restrainer holds firmly (it's dangerous to give in!) the cat will soon realize that he is helpless and usually will lie still during the entire procedure.

Pills

Force the cat's mouth open with the thumb and fingertips. Exert pressure on the corners of the mouth to open

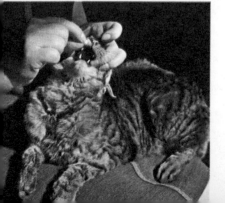

it gently. Tilt head up so you can look into it. Deposit pill as far back on the tongue as possible, then hold the mouth closed and stroke the throat to encourage swallowing. If this doesn't work, follow same procedure as above, but give the pill a little poke with your finger or the eraser-end of a pencil. A few drops of water placed on the tongue before administering the pill will help swallowing. A buttered pill also slides down more easily.

Liquid medicine

Liquids are more difficult to administer than pills. First, draw the medicine into a *plastic* bead-tipped dropper, then tilt the cat's head back and deposit liquid slowly into the deepest portion of the mouth, at the base of the tongue. If you have any doubts about this procedure, which is difficult to describe but not hard to demonstrate, ask your veterinarian to show you how.

Can Cats Transmit Disease to Humans?

The answer is yes, but the cases are very rare and the diseases are very few. Any cat owner who practices normal hygiene will rarely, if ever, be subject to any cat-transmitted disease.

For instance, ringworm could possibly be transmitted by cats, but ringworm appears in only a small percentage of cats. (Ringworm and sarcoptic mange are more often transmitted from man to cat than the other way around.) A cat owner may occasionally suffer from flea bites, but ordinarily fleas much prefer the cats to humans.

One precaution all cat owners should take — treat any cat scratch or bite with respect and an antiseptic. Otherwise, a nasty local inflammation could result, or possibly a mild fever (see page 57). A bite from a rabid cat can, of course, be extremely dangerous, but rabid cats are rarely encountered these days.

At any rate, diseases transmitted by cats are so infrequent that these words are meant as a reassurance that cats are not the disease carriers that some say they are. When you consider the amount of disease passed on from human to human, cats really turn out to be much safer friends.

Your Cat's Medicine Chest

The careful pet owner is prepared in advance for illness or injury by keeping together all items needed to nurse the stricken cat. Discuss your pet's needs with your veterinarian. Some recommended items are:

- Plastic bead medicine dropper
- Rectal thermometer
- Sterile cotton balls
- Bandages
- White (not carbolated) petroleum jelly
- Milk of magnesia tablets
- Baby oil
- Tannic acid jelly
- Antiseptic (such as Panalog)
- Carsick remedy (such as Maalox or Dramamine)
- Tranquilizers (if recommended by veterinarian)
- Aspirin (baby)
- Flea spray

Special Care for the Aging Cat

Although the average life span of the cat is around twelve years, with proper feeding and care your cat will probably pass his fifteenth birthday with you, and with luck he may still be with you when he's twenty.

Old Puss needs special care and understanding

Dear old Puss may not be as much fun when he's older, but if you love him you won't expect those bones to be as spry as a kitten's. And you'll want to keep more of an eye on him as he advances in years. For instance:

1. Watch out for erosion of tooth enamel. Have his mouth checked regularly. Those worn teeth can cause gum infections. And when Puss loses his chewers, he won't get upper plates; you'll just have to give him softer foods.
2. Notice if he is drinking an unusual amount of water. This is one of the first signs of kidney failure in an old cat. If symptoms persist, consult your veterinarian at once.
3. Watch his diet. A lean cat usually lives longer than a fat one. Those soft foods we mentioned above, along with Puss's "retirement" and inactivity, are bound to put on extra weight. That's your cue to cut the daily rations. Don't listen to his protests; he'll get used to it.
4. Many cats, like humans, gradually grow deaf with age. Allow for this in your care of him and don't expect him to come when called or to answer other verbal commands.
5. See that he doesn't get cold. Older cats sleep more. See that his favorite sleeping place is out of drafts and comfortable. Don't let him stay out all night when lower temperatures may cause sniffles or worse.

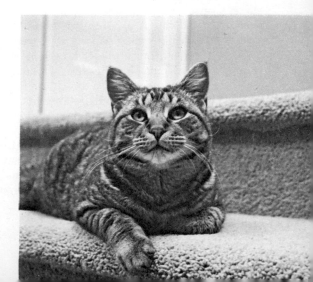

6. Keep him out of trouble. Roof-climbing is fun and natural for a young cat, but high places can mean broken bones when age takes over and joints become stiff. Puss is no longer nimble, nor is his eyesight as keen. Keep him away from the street; he's no good in a fight, so you should keep his life as peaceful as possible.

One good way to inject a little pizzazz into old Puss is to bring a new kitten into the family. He may be jealous for a few days, but he will adjust much faster to a kitten than to another adult cat. The playfulness of the small one will jog Puss's memory of what fun it used to be to chase a ping-pong ball or play leapfrog. Before you know it, your aging cat may be roughhousing with his new friend like a teenager. Great for his arteries; better yet for his morale.

When it's time to go

Despite all your loving care, the day may come when kitty is just too old, too sick, or too deaf and too blind to live happily or comfortably any more. Then it may be time to put him peacefully to rest.

Do not take on the burden of making this decision alone. Consult your trusted veterinarian, and possibly two or three. This is a painful decision to make, and if made too casually may cause you regrets.

Once the decision is made, however, do not cause yourself extra pain by hesitating. Today's animal euthanasia involves either a quick painless injection or the high altitude "euthanaire" method. Both bring permanent sleep without pain or anxiety. If your Puss is in pain, it is not love but only selfishness that would have him linger. It is time then to put him to rest, perhaps to make room in your heart and your home for some young animal, anxious for life, who may not be given such a chance unless you take him in.

5

From Here To Maternity

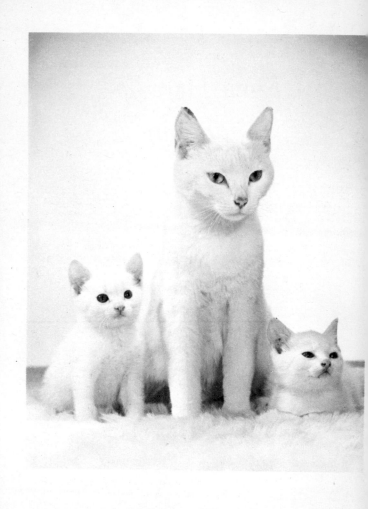

Is Sex Necessary?

Unless you plan to show or breed your cat professionally, you will have a much nicer pet if you have your cat altered. Unaltered females are restless in season — they yowl and wander. The male sprays walls and furniture, gets into fights, leaves home for days — often forever. His odor may be attractive to cats, but people don't like it at all. In fact, sprayed drapes or furniture are as effective as a smallpox sign in discouraging guests.

Altering

Altering your cat is painless and causes no change in the personality, especially if done during the first year. It can only make both male and female more gentle, placid, and homeloving. With proper diet and exercise your altered pet will not put on excess weight.

The recommended age for altering females is six months, before the first season. Males should be altered at about seven months.

Should I let her have kittens?

If you are wondering whether or not to breed your female cat, the answer is probably no. On the other hand, if you have a pedigreed pet which you plan to mate with a good stud to produce valuable kittens, you'll have no trouble finding prospective owners. But if you merely let your female wander, and allow nature to take over, you may not be able to find good homes for all of the kittens.

Too often cat owners let their females produce litter after litter, then burden their humane society with the task of finding homes. Frequently these kittens cannot be placed and must be humanely destroyed. It is estimated that there are thirty million cats in the

United States today; ten million are without homes. Don't add to the population explosion!

Don't be sentimental and think your female must know the joys of motherhood. Kittening can mean

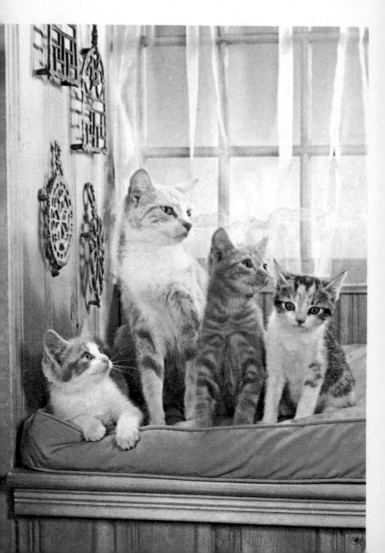

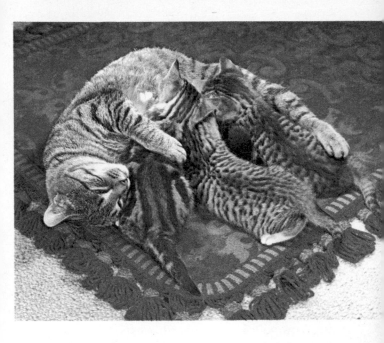

a lot of pain and hard work for her. If she never produces a litter, she'll be just as happy.

If You Opt for Maternity

If you do let your female out for moonlight strolls while she is in season, chances are that about sixty-two days later she will present you with a litter of kittens. As the day approaches, you will notice her appetite widening with her girth. Give her all the food she needs and add warm milk to her diet. The mother-to-be is not at all fragile during this period and needs her regular exercise, but handle her gently and warn the children to take extra care.

About one week before the kittens are due your cat will start searching for a nest. Unless you want her to appropriate your bottom drawer or best hat, you had better help her out by preparing a box. A large cardboard carton — roomy enough to accommodate both mother (stretched out full length) and kittens — will be suitable. Cut about three-fourths of one side out. Line the inside with shredded paper on the bottom, old towels or rags on top. Change the top towel frequently. The mother needs her nest dark to protect the eyes of the newborn kittens, so if the carton does not have a lid, put it in a dark corner or closet. Be sure to place the box out of traffic. Mother cats like quiet, and if they don't get it, will remove the kittens, one by one, to the nearest refuge.

During the kittening, stand by in case of an emergency, but do not help your queen unless she is having trouble. If she has not produced her litter within a few hours of the first signs, call the veterinarian. She may need a Caesarean.

Be sure that each kitten born is followed by a placenta. You will have to watch carefully, because the mother consumes it. If a placenta is left in the uterus it can cause metritis. If you suspect a retained placenta, call your veterinarian.

After delivery, allow the mother to clean the kittens and the box. Do not change the bedding until about three hours after she has dropped the last kitten.

Give the mother her regular food (but larger quantities or more frequently if she seems to be hungry at the time), and be sure she always has plenty of warm milk and water.

What to Do about the Kittens

In general, you need to do nothing. A mother cat takes beautiful care of her kittens and will resent your

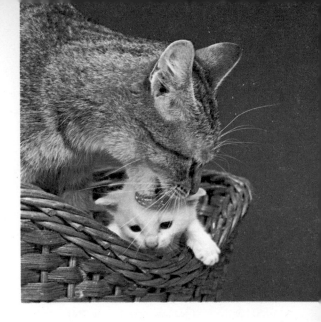

help. She will keep the kittens tidy by washing them and disposing of their waste. The kittens will be nursing almost constantly, or so it will seem, and the mother will rarely leave them except to go to her litter pan or to eat. Do not anger the mother by handling her kittens, except to help the smaller, weaker ones to get their share at the breast.

The kittens will open their eyes at about ten days. At about four weeks mother will show them how to use the sandbox.

Weaning

About one month after birth the kittens will begin getting their first set of teeth (milk teeth). You may start feeding them small but frequent meals. The mother cat will grow weary of nursing by this time and will welcome your help. Any of the Friskies canned foods, or Little Friskies moistened with Carnation Evaporated Milk, will get them off to a good start. (See Chapter 3 for tips on feeding.)

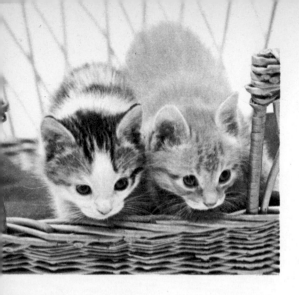

At around five weeks the kittens may leave the nursery and begin their round-eyed, stumbling exploration of the outside world. The mother cat will leave them for longer periods of time. When they are seven or eight weeks old — no sooner — they may be placed in the homes you have found for them.

Caring for orphans

Occasionally (fortunately it is not often the case), the mother cat dies during kittening or shortly thereafter. Although it is not easy to save the kittens, you can raise them successfully if you know how to take care of their needs. It is hard work, so be prepared for constant watchfulness and interrupted sleep.

If no foster mother* is available, you can feed the kittens with eye droppers or with children's doll bottles, which have tiny nipples. If any kitten refuses to lick or suck, try first putting some of the warm milk on your hand for him to lick.

*Another unspayed female cat can be turned into a mother by giving her an injection of prolactin, which will bring forth milk and actually giving her a strong motherly instinct.

You must be careful with the medicine dropper. Put only one drop at a time on the kitten's tongue. If his mouth fills with milk, he may inhale some of it, causing pneumonia.

A day-old kitten needs two to three dropperfuls, six times a day. When he weighs twelve ounces, you may feed him one once every five hours. A three-pound kitten needs about three ounces every six hours. Carnation Evaporated Milk mixed with an equal part of warm water and a small amount of Karo or honey is an excellent and inexpensive formula.

After meals, rubbing the kitten's abdomen with a warm, moist towel will replace the mother's licking and stimulate evacuation.

No homes to go to?

If your kittens have no homes to welcome them, ask friends and neighbors to help you place them. You

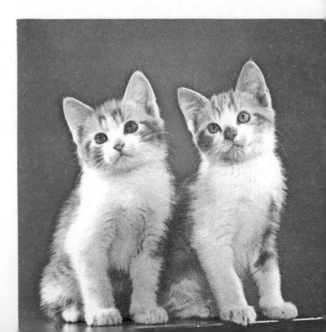

may be surprised how many people will accept a kitten. An ad in the school newspaper or on the school bulletin board is likely to attract the kind of families you would want for the kittens. If you live in a large community it is best not to advertise in the newspaper for homes for the kittens — you have no way of telling how they will be treated.

Your veterinarian, SPCA, or humane society will attempt to find homes for the kittens, but do try asking on your own first.

When placing the kittens, ask the new owners to protect the kitten with enteritis inoculations, or offer to have the kitten immunized yourself. Emphasize the need for neutering or spaying. It might also be well to give the new owners a cat booklet such as this one, available at your humane society or SPCA. You'll feel better about letting your kittens go if you know they'll receive intelligent care.

If you don't want your mother cat to have kittens again, you should have her spayed two weeks after the kittens have been weaned, or when her breasts have returned to normal. If you wait much longer, she may get pregnant again!

6

Making The Traveler At Home

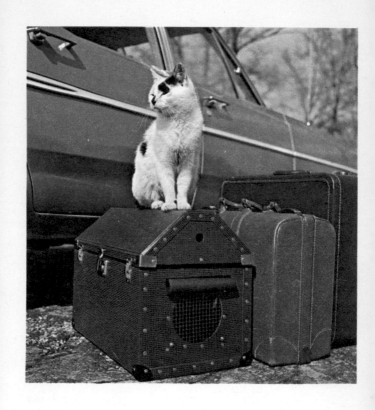

EVEN if you don't anticipate many trips with Puss, it's wise to accustom him to traveling and to be prepared with a good cat carrier. As a rule cats do not travel well, and in most cases must be confined.

The Cat Carrier

Your carrier should be large enough to contain an adult cat comfortably. It should be ventilated at one or both ends, have drop curtains, and be secured by strong latches, a lock, and a strap. It should open from the top, which should be rounded. (In case your cat is shipped, baggage cannot be stacked on a rounded carrier.)

Acquaint your cat with the carrier by letting him sleep or nap in it if he likes. Carry him about the house in it — then up the block. He'll soon feel at ease.

Automobile Travel

If properly introduced to automobile riding, most cats can learn to take it calmly, if not with pleasure. The secret lies in letting the cat get used to the car slowly. He should be allowed to sniff around the inside of the parked car until he is familiar with it. The next day try starting the motor while the cat is sitting beside you. After that you might put him in the carrier and start the motor. If all goes well, drive around the block a few times. The carrier should be placed on the floor to minimize the feeling of motion.

When and if your cat takes to automobile riding happily, he may enjoy sitting in someone's lap instead of in his carrier. If he is further protected with a collar and leash, so much the better. Never drive alone with your cat unless he is inside his carrier. He could leap toward the driver or even out the window.

Some cats get carsick. The bottom of the carrier should be lined with shredded newspapers or a towel. If traveling for any distance, you may wish to give your cat a tranquilizer, but only on your veterinarian's advice.

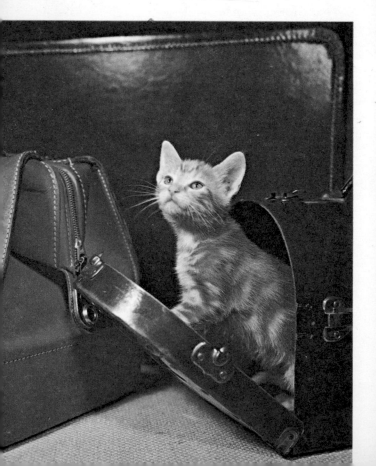

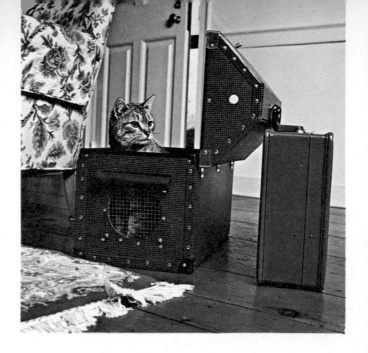

At hotels and motels

Keep your pet confined to the carrier or bathroom while you are sleeping and when you are out of the room. He could amuse himself by clawing furniture and draperies, and you will pay for his fun. Furthermore, he might leap out of the window to go exploring.

Do not condemn hotel proprietors who will not take pets. It's not that they don't like animals — only that they have too much experience with pet owners who are not as considerate as you are.

Parking

Avoid leaving your cat in a parked car. Since the windows must be left open for ventilation, you are inviting theft. It is usually easy enough to take the cat carrier with you. If you *must* leave the cat, park where it's cool, leave the wind-wings slightly open, lock the car, and hurry back.

The Bus and Subway

A cat is welcome on most public carriers, provided he's in *his* carrier. But he must be *kept* in it.

The Train

Cats in carriers are allowed on trains. If your journey is longer than twenty-four hours, you are better off putting the cat in the baggage car, where you can visit him frequently. Don't forget food and water. Dry food, like Little Friskies, is all he needs. But plenty of water is important. Make arrangements with your railroad agent in advance of the trip.

The High Seas

You will find many different types of regulations governing travel by ship. Be sure to plan in advance.

Large steamships have kennels with an attendant. Some smaller lines may permit the cat in your stateroom. (In this case, take along a small, collapsible crate — the carrier is too small for all-day confinement.) Freighters sometimes have no rules at all. If your cat is allowed to travel unconfined, be sure to take along his collar and leash.

Cats can become seasick. Ask your veterinarian what to do should this happen. Don't hesitate to ask the ship's physician for help if your cat becomes very ill.

Plane Trips

Air travel usually goes smoothly for cats, and is much the preferred method of travel. They are en route for a shorter time and are not adversely affected by the motion or the high altitude. Discuss your cat's trip with the airline officials and prepare accordingly. It may be necessary to have a health certificate and proof of rabies vaccination.

You may sometimes be permitted to take your cat (confined, of course) on the plane with you. Airlines differ in their regulations. Because the airline may allow only one cat in the cabin per trip, you should reserve space in advance.

Shipping Your Cat

Shipping a cat can be complicated and risky or fast and easy, depending on the preparations you make and your proper attention to details.

When you ship your cat, keep these points in mind:

- Label carrier "Live cat inside."
- Check with the veterinarian and procure a health certificate. File this in case of accident, neglect, or sickness incurred en route.
- Chart with your express agent a journey that has a minimum of connections and stopovers. Have some dependable person on hand at the destination to pick up the traveler promptly.
- Be sure this valuable cargo is insured.
- Try to arrange the trip when the weather is neither too warm nor too cold. See that carrier ventilation is proper for the season of the year.
- If the trip will take more than a few hours, attach food, water, and pans to the top of the crate (don't put them loose inside), with exact instructions. (Line the crate with shredded newspapers, and forget about kitty's sandbox. It will only spill.)
- Feed the cat several hours before departure so that the food will be digested before the trip starts.
- Be sure the carrier is bound by a strap. Latches can work loose.

Air shipment is the easiest way to send a cat any considerable distance. Check your airline to see if it has a reasonable flat fee for animal shipment. If not, it will be more economical to ship Air Express. When shipping by this service you may specify exactly what airline and flight you want your pet to go on. Give the recipient of your cat this information to make sure that kitty will be met at the airport.

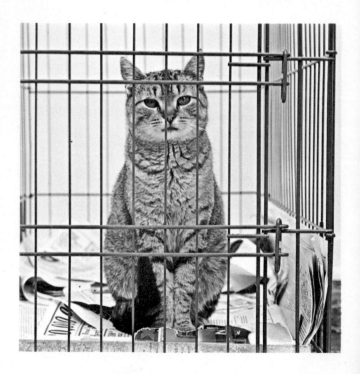

Boarding Your Pet

Don't let worries about your cat's welfare chain you to home when you wish to travel. An overprotected cat never grows up. Your cat should become used to associating with persons other than yourself so that when you leave him he can adjust to the new situation without fear.

If you are going to be gone only a very short time, you can have a responsible neighborhood child or friend come to your home to feed your cat and change the litter box. If it is a child, leave specific instructions and foods with the mother.

A kennel proprietor can also be depended on to give proper care. If your veterinarian takes in boarders, he is a good choice. His expert eye will immediately detect symptoms of an unexpected illness. The best boarding facilities for cats have outside "runs" so that kitty will not be imprisoned while you're away but can get out and stretch his legs.

7

Enjoying Your Cat

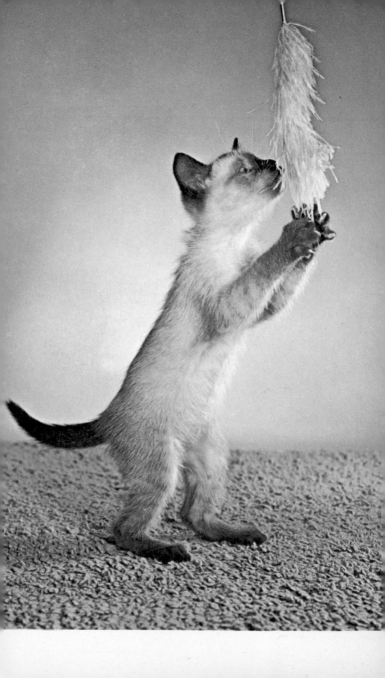

YOUR cat has so much to contribute to your life. Don't let your relationship become one of mere automatic care and acceptance. Take time to watch your cat — he's beautiful at play or in repose. Pet him often. He needs love. Get to know his beguiling ways. Read some of the many amusing and informative books or magazines on cats. They will deepen your appreciation of your pet immensely.

The Cat's Past Is as Fascinating as His Presence

In spite of the fact that cats are quite different from dogs, they were descended from the same mammal — the Miscis, a tree-dwelling animal resembling the civet. This was some fifty million years ago. From Miscis evolved the dog family, Canidae, and the cat family, Felidae, which includes lions, tigers, leopards, and jaguars. An African wildcat is believed to have been taken into southern Egypt some five thousand years ago, where the breed became domesticated.

The cat's career since then has had its ups and downs. Carved figures of cats show us that Egyptians considered them gods to be worshiped. Death was the punishment for anyone who killed a cat. Contrast this thinking with the Middle Ages, when the cat became linked with witchcraft. Both cats and their owners were supposed to be evil beings to be done away with as promptly as possible.

In the early eighteenth century, humanitarians who followed the teachings of the early Christian saint, Francis of Assisi, recognized that cats were neither divine nor diabolic — that they were the loyal friend of man and the guardian of his home and storehouse, entitled to his protection and love.

Today's small domestic cat is an omniverous digitigrade mammal (which simply means it eats flesh and nonflesh and walks on its toes), weighing from six to fifteen pounds. The life span of this lovable animal averages from twelve to fourteen years, but many cats live to be twenty or more years old because of today's enlightened care and improved nutrition.

Your Cat at Play

All felines are equipped with keen vision, acute senses of hearing and smell, plus very delicate antennae in the form of whiskers. These faculties, combined with stealth and patience, make the cat a keen hunter. Observing your pet in his supreme role of hunter, which in these days is most often just a game, will give you an appreciation for a talent that is unequaled in any other animal (except, of course, in the larger members of the cat family).

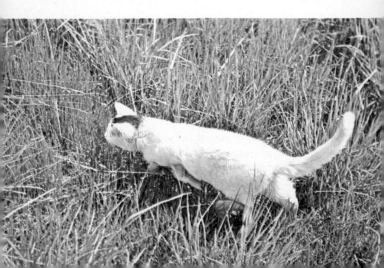

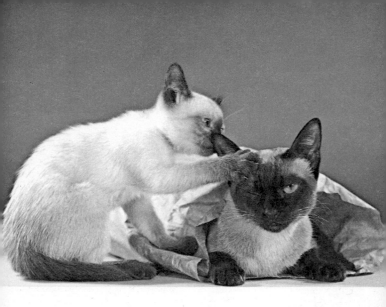

These primitive hunting instincts direct most of your cat's playtime activities. Playing is very necessary if he is to preserve that sleek muscle tone and keep his disposition at a perky par. When you play with or exercise your cat, appeal to those hunting instincts. You'll both enjoy yourselves immensely.

Boxing with your kitten is great fun, but do not let him wrestle your hand unless he learns to keep his claws in. When he grows up he may keep the clawing habit, which will be no fun at all!

A string becomes a slithering snake or lizard to a cat. Let him chase one often. But never leave a cat alone with a loose string — he can get himself into trouble by swallowing it.

A brown bag becomes a mysterious surrounding enemy, worthy of all the fight your innocent attacker has in him. Put an empty grocery bag on the kitchen floor — then watch the fun.

A spring toy (often more effective if attached to the scratching post) becomes a bird — always in flight, yet within reach. It will make your catcher joyful.

A catnip mouse not only provides easy prey for stalking but also acts as a nerve stimulant. Cats kept indoors often need this stimulation to exercise.

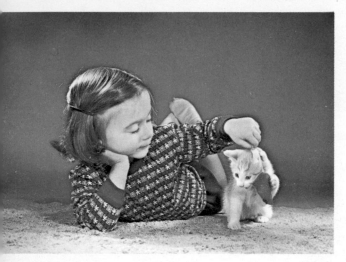

Spools and hard rubber or plastic balls also make interesting, evasive prey for the cat's paw and claw. Avoid painted objects, sharp objects, and any object small enough to be swallowed, such as a button or marble.

Get to Know His Many Moods

If you are alert, you will soon find that your cat's communication with you, whether verbal or silent, is very fluent. Several unspoken signs will keep you current with his moods. A tail fluffed out to twice its normal size means hostility. Back arched into a croquet wicket, ditto. Tail up like an exclamation point is a weather sign for self-assurance and pride. Tail down is caution. When he shakes his paw at a plate of new delicacies, he means it doesn't pass muster. If he scratches all around the dish, he is labeling it fit for burial.

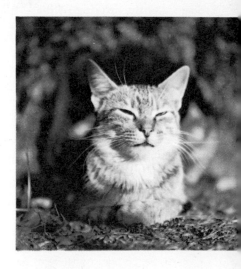

Contentment is head down, paws tucked in, tail curled around body. Meditation is the same pose but with head up, eyes like slits. Kneading a lap is love and dependency. So is a rub against the legs. (If done around mealtime Puss may be looking for tangible evidence of your love — in his dinner dish.)

Kitty's meow can mean pet me, feed me, let me in or out, pick me up or put me down, depending on when or where the meowing is done. The attentive housekeeper soon learns the private inflections of her particular Puss and can interpret her pet's speech quite accurately.

A gentle scratching under the cat's chin will almost always bring forth a rousing purr, which, of course, means unadulterated happiness.

When he brings you a "present"

Even though you might be slightly horrified the first time Puss brings in prey and deposits it proudly at your feet, try to hide your feelings and simply dispose of the offering with as little fuss as possible.

Kitty is not being "bad kitty" when he nabs that bird — he's following his hunter's instincts, and when he's successful, he compliments you with the catch, expecting lavish praise. Even if you can't work up much enthusiasm, say, "Nice kitty," and *don't* be cross.

Tricks and Training

Most cats require little training — they prefer to train themselves. Will they do tricks? Some will and some won't. But if they won't, it's not because they're stupid — it's just because they don't want to. And if you're determined to have a stunt cat, you've got to make your cat *want* to.

Cats will not perform to please you. And they cannot be coaxed with fear or trickery. If you want to work with your cat, approach him when *he* is in a mood to come to you for play or affection.

Look for some action he does naturally that is either out of the ordinary or amusing and try to get him to repeat it in conjunction with your gentle command repeated again and again. When he performs, reward him with a bit of food and flattery. He likes treats with his tricks. Be careful not to tire (or bore) the cat with practice sessions that are too long or he may grow disgusted with the whole business.

In training a cat out of a bad habit, a substitute for the habit works better than punishment. And a correction just *before* the error is more effective than after. For lack of response, a sharp, unexpected noise (like a hand clap or a newspaper swat) works better than a spank.

Come to call

It is no trick to teach your cat to respond to his name. Use it all the time when you address him, and he will look to you whenever he hears it. "Come here" is just as easy. Command your cat to do what he already wants to do — for instance, to come after a toy he has been playing with or for his dish of food. By associating the phrase "Come here, Jason!" with his action of coming to you, he will soon respond to the phrase even when the come-on enticement is not in sight.

Roll over

Teaching a cat to obey this command makes use of the same principle — doing on command something he wants to do anyway. Your cat likes to have his stomach scratched, and when you do this, he rolls over on his back. Use the words "Jason, roll over" as you stroke him, then say it while only pretending to stroke him. Repeat it again and again until the word-command can replace the action. Praise him when he obeys and offer a tidbit.

Sit up

A cat will reach for a toy or tidbit by stretching up on his hind legs. Eventually he will tire and sit back on his haunches. Then you say "Sit up!" Continue associating the word when he performs the action until the two are linked in his mind.

You may teach other lessons like "shake hands" or "lie down" by using the same technique. Learning tricks keeps your cat's mind alert and interested. But make his teaching periods short, regular, frequent — and remember — when *he's* in the mood.

8

The Well-Bred Cat – Many Shapes, Many Colors

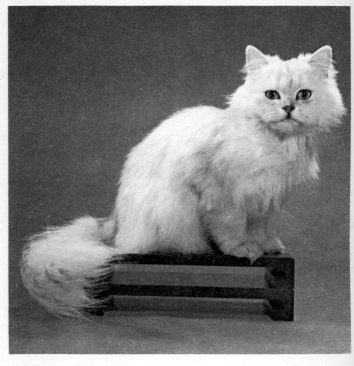

A Persian Chinchilla

Know Your Breeds

There are fat cats, trim cats, tall cats, thin cats. If your pet is just a plain, honest-to-goodness CAT, you may not know where his characteristics originate nor even care. But if he's a purebred, chances are you'll know. Following is a list of the most interesting breeds — the elite of the cat world:

The Long-haired classification, or Persian

Today about twenty to thirty varieties of colors are recognized within this classification. The Persian is known as the aristocrat of catdom, with his thick long coat (which should stand out), round head with large, wide-set eyes, short, blunt nose, and full, cobby (short, sturdy-legged) body. The heavy body and massive coat give this breed a slow-moving dignity and make it a quiet, relaxed pet, unexcelled for its decorative value. It does not like being handled a great deal, and is not as good, therefore, with small children.

Is there an Angora or isn't there?

Many people make the mistake of calling any long-haired cat an Angora, when more often than not it should properly be called a Persian.

Around the turn of the century an authority on the long-haired cat, Helen Winslow, made a distinction between the two breeds: the Angora had a silkier coat, somewhat smaller head, larger ears, slightly longer nose, and a slightly longer body and legs than the Persian. In crossbreeding, the Persian strain proved dominant, and because to most eyes there wasn't much difference, the Angora more or less disappeared as a distinct breed.

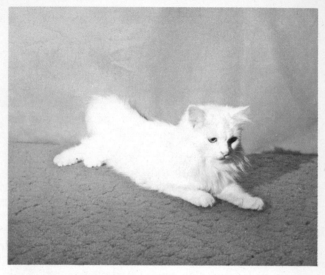

Angora (Photo by Richard Negus)

Every now and then, however, Persian breeders discover among their kittens some that do not have the round head and round eyes of the true Persian. Furthermore, cats of this Angora description are still to be seen in Turkey (Angora is the former name of Ankara), where the breed is supposed to have originated.

A California breeder recently imported several pure white Angoras and is breeding them in the hope of reviving the show standards. Although they were formerly recognized in several colors, white is the only color allowed today. Like most white cats, today's Angora is often deaf. He is remarkably intelligent, however, and adjusts easily to living with people. Some Angoras love to play in water, it is reported, and many enjoy learning simple tricks.

The Himalayan

Also known as the Long-Haired Colorpoint, the Himalayan has been produced by breeding the Persian with the Siamese. The result is what would be expected — the coat texture of the Persian, with Siamese markings. The eyes are also blue like those of the Siamese, but the body build and the shape of the face are definitely those of the long-hair — cobby body, wide face, round eyes. A Himalayan's personality also more closely resembles that of the Persian, and he is sometimes classified with that breed.

Himalayan Seal Point

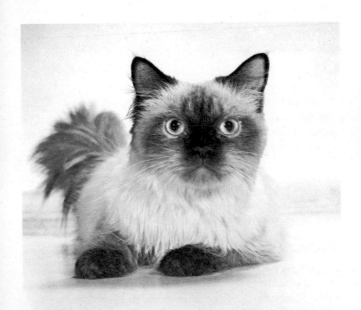

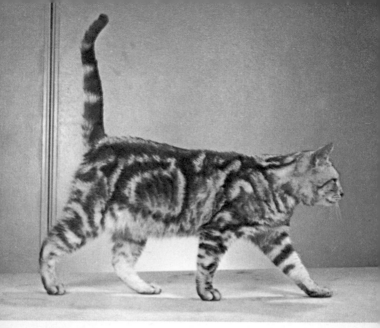

Silver Tabby

The Domestic Short-Hair

This is the most common variety of cat. Although the term is often used to describe the "alley cat" of mixed parentage, the Domestic Short-Hair is a breed in good standing today.

If the coat is not a solid color, the pattern will often be "tabby," a marking found on common and purebred cats alike. This striping is dominant, going back to the wild animal, and is not likely to disappear. The word "tabby" is derived from "Atabi," a silk ribbed with wavy lines that was produced in old Baghdad. The tabby marking comes in a variety of colors.

Breeders usually specialize in red or silver tabbies, or in Domestic Short-Hairs in solid whites, blacks, or tortoise-shells. The show standard for the Domestic Short-Hair calls for a powerfully built, cobby animal, with large eyes and a short, broad face.

The Manx

So named because some believe it came from the Isle of Man, this unusual variety of cat has no tail. The best examples actually have less than no tail — a dimple where the tail ought to be. But often stumpy or normal length tails do occur in any given litter.

Because the hind legs are long and the front legs short, the Manx hops with his round rump held high, rather like a rabbit. He wears two coats instead of one — a dense, close-lying undercoat, and a longer, soft and open top coat. These can be of any color. This amusing breed is intelligent and calm, and makes a fine, affectionate companion. The voice is soft and sweet. A pure Manx cat is rare and rather expensive. Continued pure breeding (Manx to Manx) cannot be achieved successfully; survival depends on occasional outcrosses.

Manx

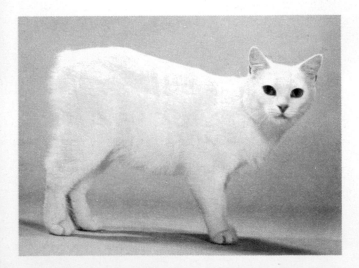

The Abyssinian

This breed has a distinctive, powerful grace, and a rather wild beauty. The ruddy or red coat is short, soft, and thick. It is ticked with black, gray, or brown. The tail is very long, and the triangular face has green, yellow, or hazel eyes.

The first of the breed seen in England (1869) was an import from Abyssinia. Authorities say the Abyssinians (often called Abys) closely resemble the sacred cats of ancient Egypt or the wild North African desert cats. The personality of an Aby retains some primitive characteristics: he is often shy and uncommunicative (he has a melodious voice but seldom uses it), exhibits much cunning and independence, and is easy to train. Unlike most other breeds, the Abyssinian is fond of water and can be an excellent swimmer.

Abyssinians are difficult to breed, produce small, predominantly male, litters, and are therefore hard to find and expensive to buy.

Abyssinian

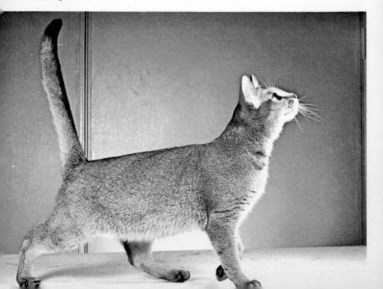

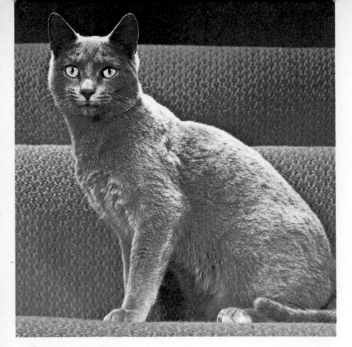

The Russian Blue

Because of his solid gray-blue coat, the Russian Blue is sometimes mistakenly called Maltese. (Maltese, not a breed at all, is merely a pretty name for a common gray alley cat.)

Russian Blues are finely boned, and have long graceful bodies and legs. Their heads are large, and they have vivid, large, wide-set eyes. The coat, unlike that of any other short-hair, does not lie smoothly. The fur is very thick and stands away from the skin. It is actually a double coat, giving the effect of glossy plush.

Short-haired blue cats of this type were supposedly brought to England by Russian sailors in the late 1800s. They have been bred in the United States since 1907, but difficulty in maintaining coat texture and color has made the Russian Blue a rare sight, even at championship shows.

If you should see a Russian Blue you would find

him quiet and gentle, but shy and hard to know. For those who do know him, his personality and antics make him appear somewhat of a clown, with a delightful, subtle sense of humor.

The Siamese

The royal cats of Siam, favorite of Siamese royalty, were at one time regarded as sacred. They were the watch cats of the temples; it is said that their loud wails warned of the approach of the enemy.

This friendly cat, by far the most popular purebred in the United States, does have an unusual voice that sounds almost as if he's talking to you. He's quick-witted and wiry, an excellent jumper and climber. Siamese cats are very affectionate. They will follow their masters like dogs and will happily walk on a leash. They are usually very sensitive and intelligent, often mischievous and highly entertaining.

The Siamese is distinguished by his remarkable

Seal Point Siamese

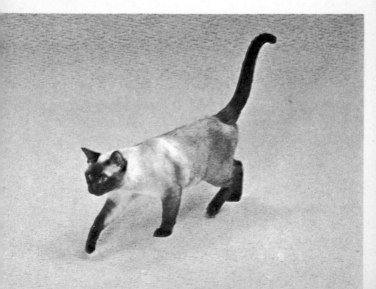

coloring. Siamese have pale fawn or cream coats, set off by "points" — dark areas on the faces, ears, feet, and tails. The eyes are a piercing sapphire blue.

There are a number of varieties of Siamese (and more are being created all the time), named according to the shade of their points. The most common is seal point, whose coat is tipped with rich seal brown. Chocolate points have a paler coat and milk-chocolate points. Blue points have areas of soft blue-gray to contrast with a coat that is just next to white; the lilac point and frost point have even paler accents.

The coat of the Siamese is glossy and fine and lies flat against the body. The body coat should contrast sharply with the points. The body is lean and graceful, with slim legs and trim paws. The tail is long and tapered and sometimes kinked, a fault in breeding. The head is narrow and tapering; the eyes should be almond-shaped and slanted toward the nose. (Those amusing cross-eyes one often sees in Siamese are also a breeding fault.)

The Burmese

This breed looks much like the Siamese, but his coat is a burnished sable-brown, sometimes shaded to a slightly lighter color on the underparts. His eyes are gold. The origin of the Burmese is mysterious. Some say that they were the beloved pets of Burmese royalty. Others say Burmese were sacred to the Indian maharajahs. Most agree that the breed arrived in this country around 1930, but how is a matter of argument. Cat authority Milan Greer says a brown male cat brought to New Orleans by a sailor was sent to Virginia Cobb in Boston, who bred this brown cat to a Siamese, inbreeding the offspring until she had purified the new line. Greer claims all Burmese in this country can trace their ancestry to this one anonymous brown cat, the likes of which have never been found in Burma.*

*Milan Greer, *The Fabulous Feline*, New York: The Dial Press, 1961

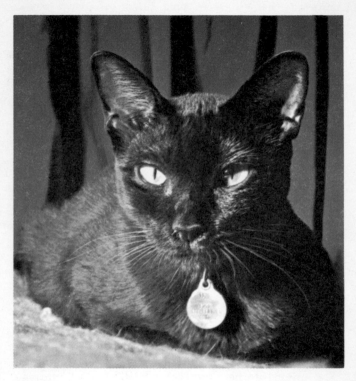

Burmese

There is *no* doubt, however, about the rapidly growing popularity of the Burmese. Their sleek brown coats are extremely attractive, and they have the intelligence and affectionate qualities of the Siamese, but are quieter and more gentle.

The Korat
The newest breed to be seen in this country, the Korat was first imported in 1959. It is still rare, although it is becoming increasingly popular in the United States.

This exotic feline is an Asian breed, and it is he, not the Siamese, that is the popular cat in Thailand (Siam) today. The Korats were first found in Korat province and are quite likely the forerunners of the blue point Siamese. Korat means "silver" in Thai, and the possession of living "silver" has been eagerly sought and jealously guarded by the Thai people.

The outstanding characteristics of this breed are its sleek, silver-blue coat and its huge expressive eyes, which are a sparkling sea-green at maturity. The coat is glossy and fine, lying close to the body. The head of the Korat is an unusual heart shape.

A medium-sized muscular cat, the Korat moves with quiet grace. He is warmly affectionate and responsive, is fond of human companionship, and can easily be taught tricks such as retrieving.

Korat

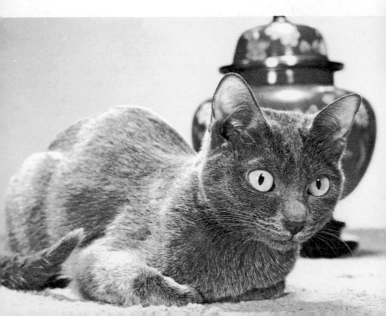

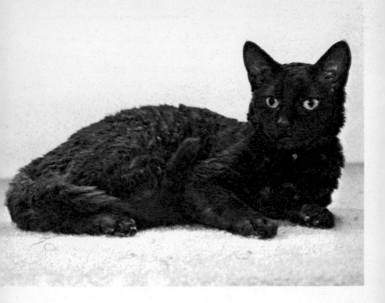

The Rex

The Rex distinguishes itself as being wavy-haired rather than long-haired or short-haired. His velvety coat of soft, curly fur is really only the undercoat and has the grace, therefore, of not shedding. Skilled breeding can now produce this practical and unusual coat in almost all the desired varieties of colors. This rare breed came into existence about 1950, and consequently is still not often seen, even in cat shows.

The body of the Rex appears delicate but feels like spring steel. His nature is very affectionate. With his nonshed coat and his loving personality, he is rapidly gaining favor as an ideal house pet.

The Maine Coon Cat

The Coon Cat is another type of long-hair worth special mention. New to cat shows, it has a long, thick coat and the temperament of the Domestic Short-Hair. The Coon Cat was so named in the mistaken belief that it was half raccoon. He has far less undercoat than the Persian and is much less inclined to suffer from mats and tangles. This is fortunate inasmuch as the Coon Cat is very active; he is an excellent fighter and "ratter."

Maine Coon Cats are rare except on Maine farms, where they are bred to keep the rat population in check. They are striking animals, coming in all colors, and in combinations with white.

Maine Coon Cat

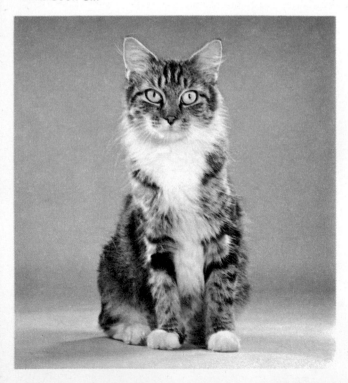

Cat Clubs

There are more than a thousand official cat clubs now on the rolls of the United Cat Clubs of America. American Cat Association, the Cat Fanciers' Association, and the Cat Federation also function in the interest of cats.

You may find it fun and interesting, even if you do not have a purebred animal, to get together with other cat lovers. Some meetings are purely social, while others feature talks on breeding and pet care. Often group members are involved in local humane projects.

For every breed of cat there are special societies, including groups dedicated to the "Short-Haired Domestic," which most of us own.

Cat Shows

Cat shows are held mainly in the fall and winter, when the cat's coat is at its best and when heat is not a problem. Often there are entries for "household pets," not necessarily purebred. If you think your

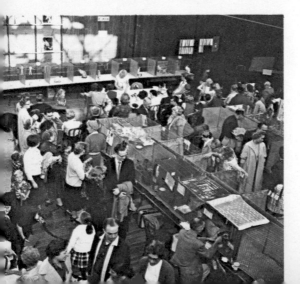

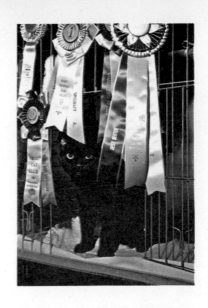

cat is extra-special in some way, you might have
fun entering. The "pet" class, of course, does not
win championships.

If you plan to show your cat, he should be regularly trained to feel at home in a cage. Several days
before showing, your cat should be bathed and have
his claws clipped close.

You can keep up with the latest in the cat world
by subscribing to such publications as *Cats Magazine*,
Cat Fancy, *National Humane Review*, or publications put out by your local SPCA or humane society.
Ask your veterinarian or check your library.

Blood Will Tell

There are now more than thirty breeds of cats,
in a multitude of accepted patterns and colors recognized by today's cat fancy (as those interested in selec-
tive breeding are called). New breeds and varieties
of breeds are being recognized all the time.

Breeding new types of cats, breeding-in new colors, or breeding patterns in or out requires tremendous knowledge on the part of the breeder, not to mention a good deal of luck.

The aim of the cat fancy is (or should be) fourfold:

1. To improve the existing physical standard for the breed.
2. To improve the health and stamina of the breed.
3. To produce new and even more desirable breeds by intelligent crossbreeding.
4. To breed and raise kittens to be pets — that is, with strong emphasis on disposition and personality.

Because interest in cat heredity is rather recent, there is still not a great deal of information about cat genetics generally available. Often breeders learn as much through experience with many litters as from encyclopedias on the subject. And there are still many non-facts about heredity being circulated, which will not stand the test of proof. You may find the following basic information on heredity interesting if you are thinking of acquiring a purebred cat.

Genes and chromosomes

The heritage of the unborn kitten is wholly contained within the sperm cell of the male and the ovum of the female. Every hereditary characteristic is determined by a pair of genes — chemical packages within the germ plasms. When the cells divide during growth, the genes congregate into strings called chromosomes. Like the genes, these too form pairs.

The male sperm and the female egg each contribute half the necessary number of chromosomes when they are joined, so that the new life gets half of its characteristics from each parent. But because certain genes are dominant over others, the offspring may resemble one parent more decidedly than the other.

We know, for instance, that the tabby gene (for striped or lined coat) is dominant over solid color, which is actually a lack of banding. Experience has proved mathematically that if you mate cats that each contain a dominant gene for tabby stripes and a recessive gene for solid color, you will get the following out of a dozen offspring: three purebred tabbies, three purebred solid colors, and six kittens with genes for both tabby and solid color. (But because striping is dominant, the probability is that nine tabbies will appear, plus three solid colored kittens.) By charting possibilities with dominant and recessive combinations in this way, inbreeding will purify lines to the desired strain.

The following characteristics can be controlled by genetic selection of dominant and recessive genes: color inheritance, markings, hair length, taillessness, eye color — as well as some undesirable traits, such as hairlessness, deafness, or polydactylism (extra toes). More and more breeders are finding that behavior traits — such as climbing ability, ratting skill, gentleness, or friendliness — can also be fostered genetically.

Inbreeding

Some believe that inbreeding (breeding brother to sister, father to daughter, mother to son) produces poor quality — weak kittens with bad personality traits. This can be true but is not necessarily so.

Because inbreeding does purify the strain, it can bring out bad characteristics, but it can also bring out good ones. If wisely done, breeding only those animals which exhibit desirable traits will definitely improve a line.

Because inbreeding will tend to make offspring smaller, occasional outcross is indicated to preserve the vigor of the line; a number of generations, however, can be inbred successfully if care is used.

In other words, inbreeding is good in itself, but should be attempted only by the knowledgeable breeder who is thoroughly familiar with the bloodline of the animals. His skill in selectivity is all-important.

Linebreeding

This type of breeding involves mating of second cousins or beyond (first cousins are considered inbred). In linebreeding, too, selectivity is important for good litters; however, since the strain is diluted, bad characteristics do not show up as dramatically.

Crossbreeding

Different breeds can be mated in order to form a new type of cat or to strengthen the existing line. By mating the progeny of a crossbreed, a pure bloodline will eventually result. The Himalayan (see page 99) is an example of a purified crossbreed. (Almost all "alley" cats are crossbreeds, too, but they have no pure bloodline.)

If you are interested in mating your purebred cat to another purebred, you should look not just at the prospective mate but also into the hereditary background to discover what recessive characteristics the cat carries. You are better off choosing a fair-to-middling offspring from a fine cat family than an excellent specimen of a fair-to-middling family. This way you are practically assured that the offspring of the cat you select will probably be better than the parent.

It is wise to choose an animal from a breeder to whom the cat's personality and adaptability are as important as show points. (You will recognize this breeder by how he treats his cats — by whether he sees them as perpetually caged show animals or as happy, well-cared-for pets.)

Once you have carefully chosen your cat's mate, you'll have to hope for luck as well as good genes. Our science of cat genetics is still in the kitten stage itself.

9

A Few Feline
Fallacies

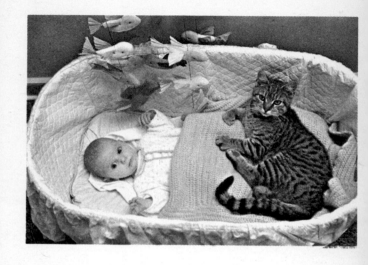

WE have tried in these pages to give you up-to-date information on what holds true for most cats. But there is a great deal being said about cats these days that is *not* true. So, in closing, we offer a few facts to dispel the myths that circulate about what certainly must be the world's most misunderstood animal. Here are some of the ridiculous statements that you as an ailurophile will have to answer to:

A Cat Will Suck a Baby's Breath

Of all the old wives' tales, this ranks among the silliest. No one seems to know how it started, but it crops up every so often. It is true that cats love cozy, warm, soft places, and a baby's crib is all of these things. Cats love to snuggle — they will curl into the hollow of one's neck for warmth and comfort. Perhaps a kitten was once found near a baby who had suffocated in its crib or died from the "Sudden Death" syndrome about which we hear so much these days. The kitten was probably blamed, even though he had nothing to do with it.

Cats Can See in the Dark

A cat has vertical pupils that expand to let him see in near-darkness. He has about thirty whiskers which help him find his way at night, even in strange surroundings. But he is not endowed with special eyesight that can enable him to see in absolute darkness.

Cats Are Surefooted and Always Land on Their Feet

Some children, believing this piece of folklore, delight in dropping Puss from heights — like out of the window — just to prove it is true. But it is more often false. Puss ends up with broken legs or neck, and it is too late to say, "It Ain't Necessarily So."

True, cats are the most agile, surefooted, graceful animals in the world — most of the time. But they can also knock over lamps, send coffee cups flying, and fall off chairs. They can end up with broken bones in short falls, especially when they are kittens.

A Cat Walks by Himself

This was a cliché before Kipling discovered it, and at best is only a half-truth. A cat's independence exists, jowl by whisker, with its opposite quality — the need to belong.

A cat needs to have friends — and the most beloved friends are not always cats. In fact, cats have been known to make friends with almost any animal alive. A cat we know well has lived for two years in perfect harmony with a white rat. She even washes him and lets him ride on her back. Another cat of our acquaintance spent many of his happiest hours romping with a bantam rooster who lived next door. Another delighted in boxing with his friend, a rabbit. Farm cats have many pals — cows, horses, goats. These relationships are proof that discrepancy in size has absolutely nothing to do with love. There is much evidence that no hostility between animals is inborn, and that even mature animals can learn to accept, without fear or anger, species other than their own.

Cats Are Cowards

Dogs are accustomed to being awarded canine Carnegies for heroism — but not many people know that cats, too, have their hours of glory.

For instance, Agatha, who saved her family from

fire by jumping on their bed. Or a cunning Siamese named Su-Ling, whose ferocious growling and tiger pounce sent a prowler scrambling. Or the courage, let alone the cunning, of the cat who scratched her sleeping mistress to save her from fire, knowing the dear, deaf lady could not hear.

There are many stories of cats scaring away poisonous reptiles, scorpions, and other unpleasant folk. In Florida, a tiny kitten was credited with alerting her mistress to the danger of a deadly coral snake.

The next time you hear someone defaming a cat's courage, come forth with one of these tales. Heroism is not confined to any one species of animal.

Cats Are Not Affectionate

The person who thinks a cat is an unloving animal never held one in his lap. (A cat, that is.) First the cat kneads gently to make the spot as soft and comfortable as possible (a happy reflex leftover from kneading his mother when he was nursing), then settles down and purrs. Whether he purrs loudly or soft-

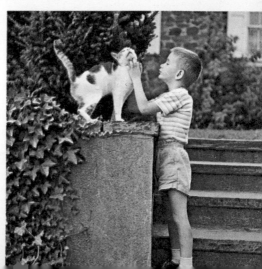

ly, it is love. A cat's affection is always subtle, like rubbing against your legs. Each cat varies in the amount of affection he wishes to pour forth, and in the ways he wishes to show it. But it's there — as long as you are receptive — and sometimes even if you're not.

Cats Prefer Places to People

This myth is closely allied to the one above. And is as untrue. For centuries cats have been moved, along with the household furnishings, from one domicile to another. If one is considerate of the cat's natural sense of dislocation and insecurity at first and lets him roam around at will to inspect the new quarters, everything will be fine.

Furthermore, tales of cats who were left behind by their owners and then found their way across unknown territory (sometimes for a thousand miles or more) to their families are legion. How they do it is one of the mysteries of science. But if places were more important than people, why would they try?

Cats Are Stupid

Physiologically, a cat's brain bears a striking resemblance to that of man — more so than any other animal's.

How do we measure intelligence in an animal? One cannot and should not play one species off against another. Cats, for example, are bored with mazes. But watch them get out of any enclosed space! They can open doors, lift latches, leap many times their own length over walls. Psychologists have noted that their ability to escape confinement is superior to that of any other animal.

Besides superb skill and strategy in stalking prey, cats have a built-in clock. They know when it is time for you to come home, and when it is time to go to bed.

Of course there are some stupid cats, just as there are some remarkable cats. Like humans, not *all* are bright.

Most often people think cats are stupid because they refuse to perform on command. But that's only because cats are smart enough to know it's beneath their dignity.

Cats Can Survive Abandonment

It is not hard to see how this legend took root. No animal lives as close to the wild state as the "domestic" cat. As far as hunting instincts are concerned, he is only a whisker away from the jungle.

Some cats, left in the woods or vacant lots by unfeeling human beings, do manage to survive. But if you have ever seen any of these cats up close, you would not recommend them as candidates for the most contented cat award. They are stringy, mangy, unkempt, and usually scared to death. Most kittens and cats abandoned in the wilds die from exposure and starvation. Cats don't really have nine lives. This is the most popular fallacy of all. Eight, maybe. But don't count on it.

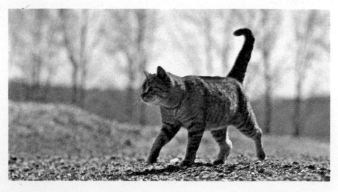

SUMMING IT ALL UP

Keep these points in mind:

• Don't let your cat's independent attitude fool you. He is totally dependent on you for proper care and love.

• Intelligent care involves taking precautions for the cat's safety and health — inoculations and consultations with your veterinarian, among other things.

• Proper feeding, which includes a varied diet he will enjoy, is all-important to the cat's appearance, disposition, and vitality.

• Cats belong at home, not on the streets, and except for exercise periods, should live and sleep in the house.

• Daily grooming, especially brushing and combing, is necessary to maintain not only a handsome coat but good health as well.

• You should be prepared with both knowledge and proper medications for your cat's illnesses or accidents — *and* be prepared to pay the cost of the proper veterinary care if necessary.

• Altering your cat, whether male or female, will make the cat a better pet. You have a serious responsibility not to let your animal breed to produce unwanted kittens.

• You should not let your pet tie you to your household. But when traveling with or boarding your pet, you have an obligation to make his life as comfortable as possible.

• You and your cat will live more happily together if you know him, enjoy him, and love him for just what he is — a superb cat.

VITAL STATISTICS
AND HEALTH RECORD

*Paste a Picture of
Your Cat in This Area*

_____

Cat's Name

OWNED BY

Name —————————————————————————————

Address———————————————————————————————

City ————————————————— *State* ————— *Zip* —————

BACKGROUND DATA

Date of Birth _____

Date Acquired _____

Breed _____

Sex _____

Color and Markings _____

Registration No. _____

Sire _____

Dam _____

Breeder _____

HEALTH RECORD AND DATA

WORMS

First Worming - Date _____

Other Wormings - Date _____

Types of Worms _____
(Identified by Veterinarian)

Medicine _____
(Prescribed by Veterinarian)

_____

VACCINATIONS

Feline Enteritis - Date _____

Rabies - Date _____

Pneumonitis - Date _____

UNSPAYED FEMALES

Dates in Season _____

Date Neutered _____

FEEDING DATA

Weaned - Age of Cat _____

Number of Feedings Daily _____

Type of Foods _____

REMINDER NOTES _____

_____

_____

_____

_____

_____

_____

_____

_____

_____

INDEX